# Jane Clarke
# Bodyfoods

## for busy people

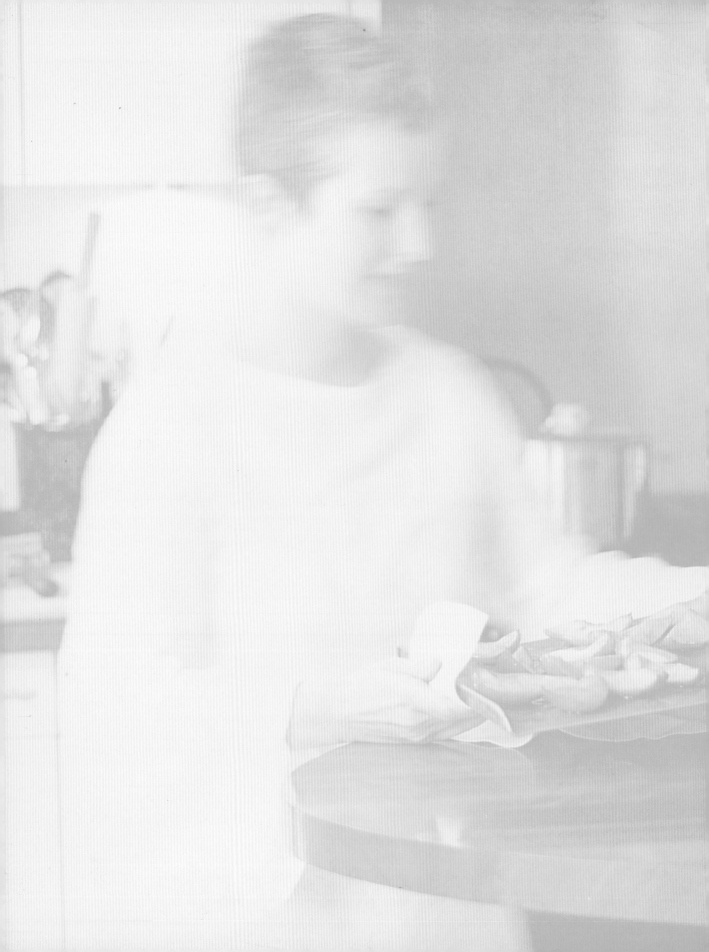

McBooks Press

Jane Clarke
# Bodyfoods

## for busy people

Published by McBooks Press 2006

First published in 2003 by
Quadrille Publishing Ltd, London

Library of Congress Cataloging-in-Publication Data

Clarke, Jane, 1966-
  Bodyfoods for busy people / by Jane Clarke.
    p. cm.
  ISBN-13: 978-1-59013-134-3 (trade pbk. : alk. paper)
  ISBN-10: 1-59013-134-7
  1. Nutrition. 2. Cookery. 3. Diet therapy. I. Title.
  TX353.C567 2006
  641.5'63--dc22
                    2006010282

Distributed to the trade by National Book Network, Inc.
15200 NBN Way, Blue Ridge Summit, PA 17214
800-462-6420

Additional copies of this book may be ordered from any bookstore or directly from McBooks Press, Inc., ID Booth Building, 520 North Meadow St., Ithaca, NY 14850. Please include $5.00 postage and handling with mail orders. New York State residents must add sales tax to total remittance (books & shipping). All McBooks Press publications can also be ordered by calling toll-free 1-888-BOOKS11 (1-888-266-5711).

Please call to request a free catalog.
Visit the McBooks Press website at www.mcbooks.com

Printed and bound in China

9 8 7 6 5 4 3 2 1

# contents

# introduction

This book was written straight from the heart. I can't recall ever having been so busy, stressed, or pushed to my limits—so much so, in fact, that this book nearly wasn't written. The reason why I've been testing my reserves to their breaking point is twofold: not only have I been busy juggling my professional goals, but above this I've been trying to realize my dream of becoming an adoptive mother.

I'm not the only person with a hectic, stressful life, however; which is why I set about pulling nutrition apart in order to discover how we can keep our bodies healthy when we're constantly hurtling from pillar to post. Leading a frantically busy life takes its toll on our bodies in the form of digestive problems, headaches, disrupted sleep patterns, and even bad-hair days—quite apart from more serious conditions like heart disease, cancer, and strokes. Although there's probably not a lot you can do to minimize the strain of living in the fast lane, it's my aim to help you to nurture and soothe your body with the food that you eat and drink. I'd like to enable you to learn the shortcuts, watch out for the pitfalls, and make healthy eating and drinking a way of life, however busy that life may be.

When we feel as though we're living on the edge, it's often the adrenaline buzz that keeps us functioning. Along with this "fight-or-flight" hormone, the body releases cortisol, a hormone whose function is to make us feel hungry enough to replenish the nutrients that the body has burned up in response to a crisis. Back in the mists of time, our ancestors' very survival depended on the ability to either stand and fight or fly from danger, but today it's usually stress that triggers the body to produce epineplatine adrenaline and, consequently, cortisol. This is why you may feel ravenous when you're under stress and why, if you respond to your hunger, you may reach for quick-fix convenience food. These are usually packed with the fat and sugar that, in the short term, may give you indigestion and headaches and, in the longer term, may cause you to become overweight. The trick to remaining healthy is firstly to understand why your body is sending out hunger signals, secondly to know which foods are best to eat in such situations, and thirdly to have those foods on hand. And that is where this book comes in.

My recipes aren't meant to be complicated, groundbreaking affairs—indeed, some of them are no more complex than how to make good toasted cheese sandwich—simply because our busy lives don't afford us the luxury of the necessary time or energy to tackle intricate cordon bleu dishes. Plenty of cookbooks provide instructions for such advanced culinary techniques, but this book combines my

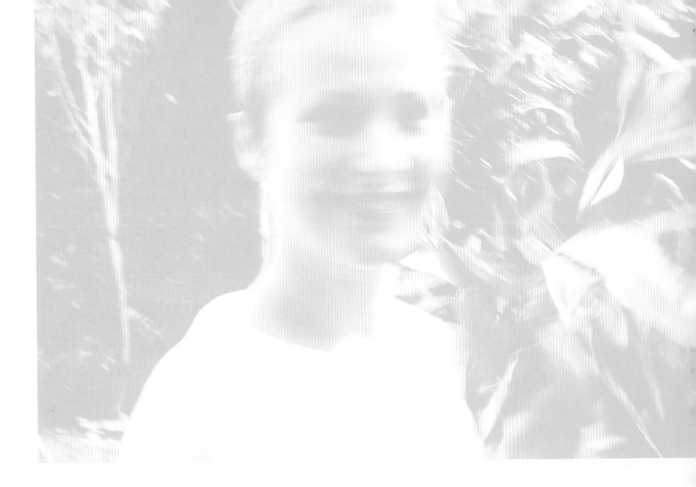

nutritional know-how with what's both practical and feasible when you're struggling to rise to the demands of a busy life. You'll find recipes for delicious and nutritious meals that can be rustled up in ten minutes flat; snacks that will provide instant energy and keep you focused; and suppers that will relax and satisfy you when you stagger through the door at the end of a tiring day, giving your body the wherewithal to wake up the next morning feeling reinvigorated and ready to deal with whatever the day throws at it. You'll also find slightly more ambitious recipes for when you have a few spare moments to get ahead.

I've also included tips on essential oils, herbal remedies, and stress-relieving exercises, because I believe that the more you do in little ways to feel good about your body, the better you're likely to treat it when it comes to eating and drinking. I suggest that you stock up with some of the remedies you're most likely to use, so that you don't have to go out of your way to hunt them down, but can just grab them when you're feeling lousy.

Jane Clarke

# bodyfoods
## basics

So much is written about healthy eating—what we should and shouldn't eat, and when and where—that you may be feeling thoroughly confused and demoralized. It's time to cut through the jargon and to focus on the essentials—the simple things you can gradually start sneaking into your time-starved schedule. If you can manage to do this, your body will slowly but surely start to feel, and look, healthier, stronger, and more capable of juggling your demands; and you will feel as if you have a life, rather than being drained by it.

# top 10 body-nourishing tips

I've put together my list of top ten body-nourishing tips that should make a real difference to your everyday health. If you can achieve all ten, nirvana potentially awaits you; but if checking off every item; on this list seems too daunting, take a day at a time to focus on meeting one target, and then move on to another tomorrow, or next week. It's best not to make any sweeping changes to your shopping, cooking, or eating routines, because the chances are that after a couple of weeks of making a concerted effort to stick to them, you'll end up reverting to your bad old ways. It's better, instead, to tweak your routine, perhaps by enjoying an energizing fresh-fruit smoothie with your breakfast or by filling your fridge with a few new ingredients to inspire you, in addition to the ones you've been buying for years. It's fundamental to remember that the secret of enjoying a healthy lifestyle lies in staying positive about your body and not beating yourself up about food. Negativity seems to attract unhealthful food and crazy ideas. Just bear in mind that your body can work only with the fuel you feed it.

1 Drink around 5 pints of water every day, staggered throughout the day to help your body hold onto it. If a dehydrated body receives an extra 1¼ pints of water, it will repay you by giving you an extra 20 percent of energy!

2 Keep your energy constant, and give your body all of the antioxidants it needs to stay young and healthy by eating five succulent fresh fruits a day.

3 Treat your body to a health-giving supply of fiber and antioxidants by having vegetables twice a day, be they raw, steamed, roasted, stir-fried, or even packaged salad greens or frozen vegetables.

4 Rather than adding salt, which can raise your blood pressure and aggravate fluid retention, use fresh herbs and spices, such as basil, parsley, dill, freshly ground black pepper, lemongrass, and garlic, to enhance food's natural flavors.

5 An aromatic cup of coffee or tea can be life enhancing, as long as it's a good-quality beverage that you really savor. But don't have more than two or three cups a day; too much caffeine aggravates stress, energy swings, headaches, and anxiety, as well as inhibiting your body's absorption of essential nutrients like calcium and iron.

6 Before drinking alcohol, either prepare your stomach by having something to eat—even if only a banana —or wait until you've sat down to enjoy a meal. You'll also sleep more soundly and feel better the next day if you drink a couple of glasses of water for every glass of wine.

7 Twice a day, eat protein-rich foods, like chicken, fish (especially oily fish), seafood, eggs (which don't raise blood-cholesterol levels), lean meat, or legumes. All of these will boost your energy levels and improve your concentration. Protein-rich foods also keep you satisfied for longer.

8 Do your skin, bones, and taste buds a favor by ditching processed foods labeled "low-fat" and "low-sugar." Small amounts of full-fat butter, cream, cheese, and even chocolate are much more delicious, as well as more healthful, than their overprocessed counterparts.

9 Maintain the strength of your bones, blood, and immune system by having some calcium-rich and iron-rich foods every day. Calcium is found easily in milk (and skim milk contains just as much calcium as whole milk), cheese, yogurt (ideally organic, containing live, probiotic cultures), green, leafy vegetables, small-boned fish, like sardines, tahini, and dried apricots and figs. Iron-rich foods include dark-green, leafy vegetables, legumes, dried fruits, whole grains, eggs, cashew nuts, and lean red meat.

10 Eat whole-grain foods every day. These help to nurture the growth of positive bacteria in the gut, which in turn produce substances (such as butyrates) that reduce the signs of aging, as well as the risk of developing cancer, heart disease, and other life-threatening conditions. Choose from whole-grain cereals, oats, whole-wheat bread (rather than brown, which may contain no more fiber than white bread, but is dyed to mislead you), wholegrain rice, or pasta. Other great fiber-packed foods are legumes, including lentils.

# energize your body with 5 pints of water a day

Not only are you what you eat; you are also what you drink. Drinking plenty of water is one of the most important ways of keeping your body feeling, performing, and looking well. When I've hit my target of 5 pints a day, I feel focused and energetic, my skin looks supple and rosy, my eyes sparkle, I feel in control of my digestive system; the list is endless.

Water benefits your body in countless ways. Rehydrating a dehydrated body will certainly give you more energy. Particularly when drunk at mealtimes, water enables your body to digest food more efficiently, increasing its ability to glean nutrients from the food, helping your stomach to gauge when you've eaten enough, and assisting the bowel in getting rid of waste products. It also improves your body's ability to deal with the sugar and salt in food, so that it doesn't retain too much of these potentially health-damaging substances. Indeed, many people find that drinking plenty of water reduces fluid retention (especially premenstrual puffiness in the fingers, feet, and breasts), as well as cushioning unsettling swings in blood-sugar levels.

I urge you to drink 5 pints of water a day, staggered over the course of the day—try sipping one glass every hour—to enable your kidneys to hold onto it better. The best way of checking whether your body's sufficiently hydrated is to glance at your urine, which should be very pale in color, not dark yellow.

## tap or bottled? carbonated or non-carbonated?

In terms of their ability to hydrate your body, there's no difference between tap and bottled water, carbonated and non-carbonated. In terms of their health benefits, the bacterial and chemical composition of tap water is generally subject to tighter regulations, which makes it a surer bet and thousands of times cheaper than bottled water. If you prefer bottled water, opt for one labeled "natural mineral water" because this type is subject to the strictest regulations; and make sure you drink it within twenty-four hours of opening to prevent the proliferation of bacteria. You may be surprised at how much salt some bottled waters contain: too much salt is bad for you, so be aware of what you are consuming. Similarly, although some flavored waters offer a palatable change from plain water, note that many contain unhealthful additives.

## the natural alternative

Although some nutritionists say that drinking 5 pints of any type of fluid will keep you hydrated, I have reservations about flooding your body with caffeine-containing coffee, tea, cola, and chocolate or additive- and preservative-laden sweet, carbonated and artificial fruit drinks, because they all have potential downsides. Drinking one or two caffeine- or sugar-loaded drinks a day won't do too much damage, but any more than this and you risk aggrevating mood swings and imbalanced energy levels (see pages 24–5). It's far healthier to rely on water and caffeine-free herbal teas.

## herbal teas to hit the spot

Aromatic herbal tea bags are a more practical option than carrying around loose-leaf tea; stash some in your handbag, briefcase, or desk drawer for when you crave a hot drink, but not a caffeine hit. Herbal teas are best enjoyed straight, without milk or sugar. Each herb has its own distinctive taste, and some alleviate specific ailments. Here are some of my favorites, which, besides tasting great, all have magical qualities to offer.

Camomile alleviates digestive disorders, nervous tension, and irritability, helping you to unwind. It can reduce phlegm and ease hay fever, and for some women reduces the effects of morning sickness.

Cinnamon traditionally alleviates colds, flu, and digestive problems. It also has the power to settle a stomach first thing in the morning. A great builder-upper when you're feeling weak and wan.

Echinacea stimulates the immune system and raises the body's resistance to bacterial and viral infections. An antibiotic and allergy reliever, it is particularly good for clearing up problem skin.

Elderflower soothes and clears chesty coughs, colds, and flu. It relieves wheezy and asthmatic chests, the symptoms of hay fever, and rhinitis. It fights fevers and builds up the immune system.

Fennel relieves bloating, soothes stomach pain, and treats upset stomachs, indigestion, and gas. It also stimulates the appetite and calms inflamed joints.

Ginger alleviates morning sickness, colds, and digestive complaints, such as wind, colic, indigestion, and constipation.

Green tea contains an army of antioxidants, which help to reduce free-radical damage. It has as much caffeine as black tea, so if you prefer to avoid caffeine, opt for another herbal tea.

Jasmine relieves tension like no other herbal tea; it calms, soothes, and has also been found to lift gloomy moods.

Lemon verbena calms upset moods and uncomfortable digestive systems, which makes it especially good for stressed-out bodies. Some people find its lemon oil helps to lift melancholy.

Nettle relieves the symptoms of hay fever, arthritic inflammation, and pain, and corrects anemia. Somewhat surprisingly, when it's applied externally, it soothes nettle rash and insect bites.

Peppermint calms the digestion, so is particularly useful when suffering from gas. It also helps to soothe colicky babies.

Saint-John's-wort destresses and is the best-known herbal remedy that naturally lifts moods. It also provides relief from tired, aching muscles and joints.

Thyme alleviates sinus pain and mild asthma, clears blocked noses, and soothes chesty coughs.

Vervain helps treat premenstrual syndrome, stress, and nervous exhausion. It also aids digestion, bolsters the nervous system, relieves headaches and migraines, and speeds recuperation from illness.

# use the power of antioxidants with five fruits a day

Fruits are packed with antioxidants (a group of powerful nutrients that fight the damage to your body caused by free radicals), including vitamin C, beta carotene, vitamin E, vitamin B complex, folic acid, and magnesium. Besides warding off such serious illnesses as cancer and heart disease, building up an internal store of fruit-derived antioxidants will help to fight the colds and bugs to which you're constantly exposed, particularly in air-conditioned offices, and are most susceptible to when tired or stressed.

The benefits of incorporating fruit in your diet are manifold: besides helping your body to absorb essential minerals, like iron, fruits such as bananas, oranges, and dried fruits are rich in potassium, a mineral that works with sodium to regulate your body's fluid balance, thereby reducing fluid retention— deflating puffy ankles, fingers, and the area around the eyes—and lowering blood pressure. Strawberries contain elegiac acid, which works to destroy the damaging hydrocarbons in cigarettes. Freshly juiced oranges contain folic acid, a powerful antioxidant thought to reduce the incidence of heart disease, retard the aging process, and limit the risk of neural-tube defects in babies. Cranberries contain anthocyanins, substances that discourage harmful bacteria from sticking to, and damaging, the body's cells, causing painful conditions like cystitis and gum disease, while papayas contain rutin, which helps to maintain strong blood vessels, especially the tiny ones running through the skin, thereby warding off unsightly thread veins.

## instant ways to your daily antioxidants

Although supplement manufacturers suggest that we can remain healthy only if we swallow their products, when it comes to antioxidants like vitamin C, this is not so. Unless you smoke, in which case boost your vitamin C levels with a 2,000mg supplement, you can easily meet your daily requirement of 60mg of vitamin C by eating plenty of fruit. Provide your body with all of the vitamins and other antioxidants it needs, without resorting to supplements, by tucking into five servings of fruit a day. A serving constitutes one orange, apple, banana, or grapefruit; approximately 1 cup of strawberries, blueberries, cherries, or other small fruits; a good-sized slice of melon, mango, or pineapple; a handful of dried apricots, prunes, or other dried fruits; and half a cup of freshly squeezed fruit juice.

Aim to eat five servings of fruit a day to provide your body with all the antioxidants and fiber it needs. Although I've specified fruit, don't worry if you end up averaging three servings of fruit and two of vegetables. What could be easier, or more delicious? Start the day with my Blueberry and Blood Orange Vitamin C-boosting Smoothie, and you'll reach your antioxidants target in a few energizing gulps.

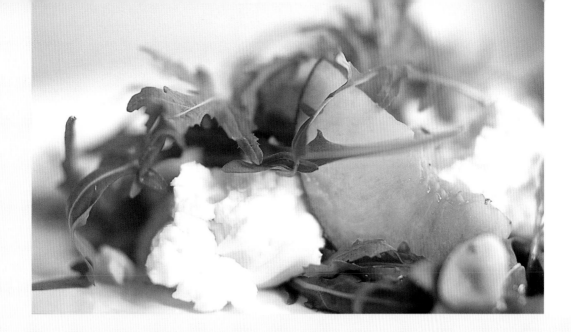

## BLUEBERRY AND BLOOD ORANGE VITAMIN C-BOOSTING SMOOTHIE (SERVES 1)

*A quick and easy way to glean an array of antioxidants in one hit. Experiment by mixing different fruits: bananas with yogurt give a creamy consistency, while citrus fruits make a juicelike smoothie.*

Juice 2 medium-sized blood oranges using a hand-held juicer, then transfer to a blender or food processor. Add 3/4 cup blueberries, 1 medium-size banana, and 3 Tbs. organic natural yogurt. Blend until smooth. Drink at once.

## PEACH AND GOAT CHEESE SALAD WITH ROASTED HAZELNUTS (SERVES 1–2)

*Cheese and fruit are one of life's great combinations (and my favorite simple supper). Virtually any cheese goes well with fruits, but goat cheese is a winner. Try also ricotta, mozzarella, or a hard cheese like cheddar or Comté.*

**For the salad**
4 cups arugula leaves
5 oz. young, soft goat cheese
4 ripe peaches, sliced into eighths
freshly ground black pepper and sea salt
scant 1/4 cup unsalted hazelnuts, broken
  into pieces

**For the dressing**
4 Tbs. virgin olive oil
2 Tbs. hazelnut oil
2 Tbs. fresh lemon juice
2 Tbs. balsamic vinegar
1/2 tsp. Dijon mustard
1/2 tsp. sugar

Put the arugula leaves into a serving bowl. Slice or crumble the goat cheese over the leaves. Add the peaches. Place the dressing ingredients in a screw-top jar. Screw the lid on tightly and shake vigorously. Drizzle a little dressing over the salad (refrigerate the rest for future use), and season with plenty of freshly ground black pepper and a little sea salt. Sprinkle the hazelnuts on top.

## fruity facts

Fruits are naturally sweet, so they satisfy any sugar craving. Fruits also contain fiber, which helps to keep your digestive system working smoothly, stimulates the production of butyrates and other cancer-fighting substances, and encourages the liver to produce high-density lipoprotein ("good" cholesterol), thereby warding off heart disease. Fiber slows down the rate at which sugar is absorbed, so a piece of fruit combining fiber and fructose gives you a sustained energy infusion without your later feeling shaky and low.

## Isn't too much fruit fattening?

Rest assured: a couple of bananas, a small bunch of grapes, or a few slices of pineapple as part of your five daily portions won't pile on the pounds. Although bananas, grapes, and pineapples, along with other particularly sweet fruits, contain more fructose than their tarter fellows, their fiber content enables it to be absorbed slowly, so you shouldn't gain any weight.

## Is organic fruit more healthful than non-organic?

I think so. Not only is organic fruit free from pesticides, antibiotics, and chemical residues, but ongoing studies suggest it contains higher levels of vitamins and minerals than nonorganic fruit. Admittedly, organic produce is more expensive, so if you're on a budget, split your money between organic and nonorganic fruit. If you don't have the time to shop around, reduce the hassle factor: try a home-delivery organic box scheme or an online supermarket delivery.

## raw or cooked?

Fresh, raw fruits usually contain the highest levels of vitamins and minerals, which makes them a more healthful option than cooked fruits. Yet vitamins and minerals are useful only if your body can absorb them, and if raw fruits send you dashing to the john or cause pain and bloating, cooked fruits, such as poached pears, baked peaches or apples, or my Fruit Confit in Spiced Syrup, may give your digestion a less rough ride.

## canned, frozen, or dried?

Although canned fruit retains its high beta carotene content, the heat-treating process involved in canning does reduce the fruit's natural vitamin C. That being said, some food manufacturers replace the lost vitamin C with its supplementary equivalent, which is just as good for you. A plus is that canned fruits are easier for people with sensitive digestive systems to tolerate. Choose natural fruits in juice, not syrup. Frozen fruits, especially berries, are very versatile, combining practicality with as many vitamins and minerals as fresh fruits. Defrost them, as needed, to make smoothies and add to cereals, crisps, and compotes. Dried fruits are great energizers, but be warned that eating too many may give you an uncomfortable sugar high and possibly cause bloating. If you find dried fruits a little hard to digest, try soaking them in water overnight. Choose organic dried fruits that contain no added sulfur dioxide (labeled as $SO_2$).

## ICY PAPAYA WITH LIME YOGURT CREAM (SERVES 4)

*Papaya is wonderful frozen, especially when teamed with tangy lime, but you could use mango or melon instead. This recipe takes only 10 minutes to put together. I like to run a bath once I've put the papaya in the freezer—good time management!*

1 large papaya, deseeded, peeled
  and sliced lengthwise
1¼ cups Greek-style natural yogurt
finely grated zest and juice of 2 limes

2 pieces of preserved ginger in syrup, finely
  chopped, plus 4 Tbs. of the syrup
⅝ cup pistachio nuts, chopped

Scatter the papaya slices over a sheet of waxed paper, cover them with another sheet, and place the "envelope" in the freezer for at least 1 hour. Meanwhile, spoon the yogurt into a large bowl, and stir in the lime zest and juice, ginger, and ginger syrup (if you prefer the cream sweeter, add a little more syrup). Divide the yogurt cream among four glasses, then refrigerate until you're ready to eat. Before serving, decorate with pistachio nuts and icy papaya strips.

## FRUIT CONFIT IN SPICED SYRUP (SERVES 2–4)

*Combining the fruit with a spiced syrup gives you a dessert to raise your energy levels.*

4⅜ cups fine granulated sugar
mixture of spices, including 4 cloves,
  2 cinnamon sticks, 3 star anise fruits, and
  a few mustard seeds, crushed
1 vanilla bean

2 oranges, peeled and cut into eighths
2 clementines, peeled and cut into eighths
1 pink grapefruit, peeled and cut into eighths
1 pineapple, peeled, cored, and cut into chunks
1 or 2 star fruits, sliced

In a heavy-bottomed, stainless-steel saucepan, bring 1 quart water to the boil with the sugar, then add the spices and vanilla. Cook over a medium heat for 5–10 minutes. Lower the fruits into the syrup and simmer for 1½–2 hours or until the syrup is translucent. Heat the broiler to a medium-high heat. Lay the fruits on a broiler pan lined with foil, sprinkle with extra sugar, and broil until golden brown. Transfer to a serving plate. Reduce the syrup until it's thick, but not gluey, and drizzle over the fruits before serving.

## RUBY ORANGE AND RASPBERRY SALAD (SERVES 2)

*Tangy raspberries with orange and mint will kick-start your taste buds and tempt a jaded palate.*

Using a sharp knife, remove the peel and pith from 4 large ruby oranges, then slice thinly through the segments. Arrange the orange slices on a serving plate with 2½ cups raspberries. Finely chop 2 fresh mint leaves, then sprinkle over the fruit. Refrigerate for a couple of hours before serving.

# learn to love
# life-enhancing vegetables

It's widely known that vegetarians tend to live longer, have fewer heart attacks, and are less prone to developing cancer than meateaters. This is not just because their diets contain far fewer—if any—saturated animal fats. No, the protective magic lies primarily in the high quantity of vegetables and fruits that their diets contain. If you are a meateater, the good news is that regularly eating lots of vegetables and fruits can similarly cut your risk of developing most types of cancer by as much as 75 percent.

Nutritionists worship vegetables because they are bursting with beneficial nutrients. These include the antioxidant vitamins A, C, and E; the carotenoids and flavonoids (themselves antioxidants), which contain compounds that stimulate the body to produce more of its own antioxidant enzymes; and the minerals iron, calcium, magnesium, and selenium, which also protect from disease.

To derive the maximum benefit from vegetables, buy and eat those (preferably organic, see page 16) that are at their freshest and ripest, because their antioxidant content increases as part of the ripening process. Wash your vegetables well, but avoid peeling them if you can, because their skins contain the highest concentration of antioxidants.

## fiber providers

Plant foods also provide us with fiber—substances that are not easily absorbed by the gut and that pass undigested through the digestive system into the bowel, where they are fermented by bacteria. Two types of fiber are present in vegetables and fruits—insoluble and soluble—and although most vegetables contain both types, the proportions vary.

All plants contain insoluble fiber (mainly in the form of the cellulose that makes up the walls of the plant's cells), which encourages the gut to keep moving efficiently, thereby averting constipation and hemorrhoids, and sometimes even diverticulitis, irritable-bowel syndrome, and cancer, because once within the digestive system, the fiber swells in the presence of water and bulks out our stools, making them softer and easier to pass. By swelling when it comes into contact with water, insoluble fiber also stimulates stretch receptors in the stomach lining to send signals to the hypothalamus, the part of the brain that registers satiety, which is why teaming celery with cheese will make you feel more satisfied than eating cheese by itself. Soluble fiber, which is found in vegetables, legumes, and oats, reduces low-density lipoprotein levels (LDL or "bad cholesterol") and helps to maintain steady blood-sugar levels. This makes an oatcake one of the most energizing of snacks (see My Favorite Oatcakes on page 80), especially if you drink some water, because although some oatcakes contain sugar, its soluble fiber reduces its impact on your blood-sugar level.

Certain plant foods offer additional benefits to health. Walnuts, almonds, and hazelnuts contain omega-6 fatty acids, which both lower levels of blood cholesterol (see pages 124–5) and improve the ratio of "good" cholesterol (high-density lipoprotein, or HDL) to "bad" cholesterol (LDL). Onions, kale, and broccoli contain quercetin, a flavonoid that may protect against the production within the body of cholesterol-oxidation products (COPS), which are toxic to the arteries and make them more likely to attract cholesterol, which furs them up. For their part, artichokes and oats increase levels of HDL and reduce heart-damaging homocysteine levels. Vegetables like Belgian endive, Jerusalem artichokes, leeks, and onions furthermore encourage the growth of healthy bacteria within the gut, inhibiting disease-causing bacteria from proliferating and producing toxins (again, the fresher the vegetable, the higher its prebiotic content).

## the serving problem

It is generally accepted that five servings of vegetables or fruits a day provide your body with all of the vitamins it needs. Meeting this daily target may initially seem daunting, but if you break the day into segments, it'll seem much more achievable. Have a freshly squeezed juice for breakfast, perhaps with a piece of fresh fruit (or save that for a mid-morning snack), a salad with your lunch, some fruit as a late-afternoon snack and vegetables with your supper, for example, and you'll have hit the five-portion mark. I love vegetables, and include them in both of my main daily meals, also increasing my five servings a day with extra legumes, such as baked beans or chickpeas (garbanzoos).

It's worth taking a few moments to work out how much of a particular vegetable you should have if it is to count as a portion—don't kid yourself that a small stalk of celery dipped in hummus is enough! Don't become obsessed with measuring your vegetables, but keep the following guidelines in mind. A serving of raw salad greens should measure at least 1 cup; a serving of cooked vegetables should measure at least ½ cup (in the case of green beans or root vegetables, such as carrots or beets, these should be chopped or sliced before measuring); a serving of vegetable juice should measure ¾ cup. Bear in mind that five servings or portions a day (of fruit and vegetables) are considered the minimum; eat more if you can.

It's best to have a varied vegetable intake, partly to prevent yourself from becoming bored with just two or three staples, partly to give your body as wide a range of vitamins and minerals as possible, and partly to boost your body's levels of a specific nutrient if you feel it necessary (vegetables tend to be rich in different types of nutrient: carrots in beta carotene and spinach in iron, for instance). Finally, if practicality is important to you, as it is to me, you'll be pleased to hear that frozen vegetables can be just as nutritious as their fresh counterparts.

# add some extra spice to your life

The less salt you eat, the better. Salt doesn't just have a negative effect on people with high blood pressure; it increases bone loss, aggravates fluid retention, and irritates the kidneys. Yet sometimes a little salt is necessary in order for food to be flavorsome; otherwise your brain doesn't recognize and enjoy the experience. Therefore, concentrate on using fresh herbs and spices, and then, if you still need to add flavor, use a little good-quality sea salt. Ditch the habit of salting food before you've tasted it.

## MARINATED ZUCCHINI AND CILANTRO SALAD (SERVES 2)

*I gleaned this idea from a vegetarian café in Paris and find it's one of the best ways to serve zucchini, which can otherwise seem a little on the dull side.*

1 heaped tsp. coriander seeds

3 Tbs. olive oil

1 medium-sized red onion, finely chopped

1 garlic clove, crushed

6 black peppercorns

1 Tbs. white wine vinegar

$3/8$ cup white wine

1 small lemon

12 oz. small zucchini, sliced into 1-in. diagonal
  or round chunks

1 very ripe tomato, skinned and chopped

1 Tbs. chopped fresh cilantro leaves

Place a skillet pan over a medium heat. When hot, add the coriander seeds and dry-roast them for 1–2 minutes, shaking the pan from time to time. As soon as the seeds start to jump, remove from the heat and tip into a mortar. Return the pan to the heat. Add 2 Tbsp. of the olive oil, the onion, and the garlic clove. Let the onion and garlic soften for about 10 minutes. Add the peppercorns to the mortar and crush. Pour the white-wine vinegar and white wine into the onion mixture, and then add the crushed coriander and peppercorns, and the lemon juice, and season with a little sea salt. Bring the mixture to simmering point, turn down the heat, and simmer gently for 5 minutes. Add the zucchini to the sauce, together with the tomato. Stir well, cover, and simmer over a gentle heat for about 15 minutes, or until the zucchini are tender but still retain some bite. Carefully stir in the cilantro leaves. Transfer the salad to a serving dish to cool, cover, and chill until you need it (but don't forget to bring it back to room temperature, which takes about 30 minutes, before serving). To serve, drizzle the salad with the remaining olive oil, and garnish it with a few sprigs of fresh cilantro.

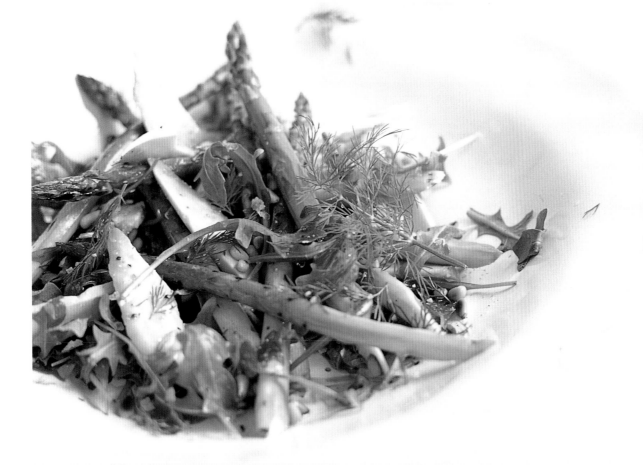

## ASPARAGUS, AVOCADO, PINE NUT, AND DILL SALAD (SERVES 2)

*This simple, delicately flavored salad would make an ideal appetizer for a special meal, particularly in summer—the asparagus season!*

9 oz. asparagus, trimmed

olive oil, for brushing

1 handful of arugula

1 ripe avocado, stoned and sliced

1 handful of pine nuts, roasted

*For the dressing*

2 Tbs. olive oil

1 Tbs. chopped, fresh dill

juice of 1 lime

Heat the broiler to medium. Trim the asparagus, and then, using a vegetable peeler, strip away 2 in. of the skin from each stalk. Lay the asparagus on a broiler pan in a single layer, and brush lightly with a little olive oil. Broil for 5—6 minutes, turning occasionally, until tender and light golden in parts. Sprinkle some freshly ground black pepper and a little sea salt on top, then leave to cool slightly. Mix together all the dressing ingredients. Season to taste. Arrange the asparagus on serving plates and top with the arugula and avocado. Drizzle the dressing over, sprinkle with pine nuts, and serve immediately.

## FRESH BORLOTTI BEANS WITH THYME (SERVES 4)

*You may ask why, if time is short, I've included a slow-cook bean recipe; but once you've assembled the ingredients, which takes roughly 10 minutes, you can relax before returning an hour later. Borlotti beans are also known as cranberry beans or french beans. If you can't find borlotti beans, use pinto beans instead.*

2¼ lb. fresh borlotti beans, podded

6 ripe medium-sized vine tomatoes

2 small garlic cloves, whole

1 bunch of fresh thyme

½ cup extra-virgin olive oil

Heat the oven to 400°. Place the beans in a terracotta casserole dish large enough for the beans to take up half of its depth. Add the tomatoes, garlic, and thyme. Pour in cold water (or cold chicken or vegetable stock) until there is about ¼ in. water between the top of the beans and the water level. Drizzle the extra-virgin olive oil on top. Place a piece of aluminum foil over the dish, tucking in the edges to seal. Make a small hole in the middle of the foil to allow the steam to escape as the beans cook. Place in the oven and cook for approximately 1 hour, during which time the liquid will be absorbed by the beans, which will soak up the flavors of the olive oil, tomatoes, and thyme. Remove from the oven and gently stir the beans, which should now look delicious and creamy. Season with lots of freshly ground black pepper and a little sea salt, and drizzle a dash of extra-virgin olive oil over the top.

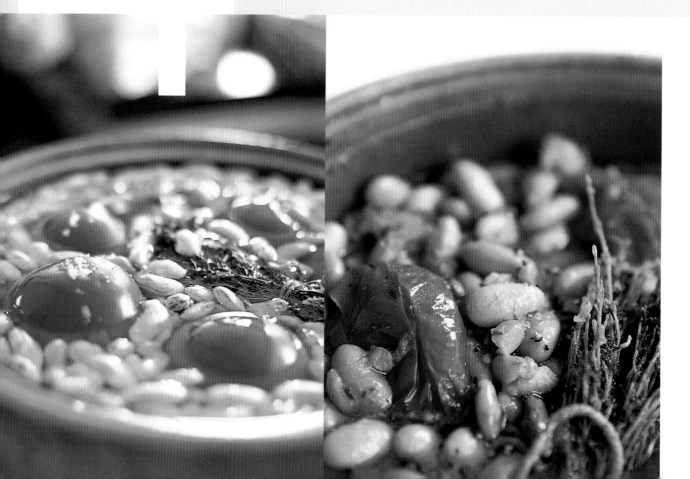

## ROASTED BEET AND CHICKEN SALAD (SERVES 4)

12 small, fresh beets, thoroughly washed

1/4 cup olive oil

4 cups washed and dried mixed salad greens
  (such as watercress and Belgian endive)

1 small bunch of fresh tarragon leaves

2 ripe avocados, peeled, stoned, and sliced

9 oz. roast chicken meat, cut into
  small pieces

*For the dressing*

1 Tbs. balsamic vinegar

1/4 tsp. Dijon mustard

scant 1/2 cup olive oil

Heat the oven to 375°. Trim the beets, reserving the young leaves to add to the salad. Place the beets in a roasting pan, drizzle with the olive oil, and sprinkle with some freshly ground black pepper and a little sea salt. Roast in the oven for approximately 40–60 minutes, or until they are slightly crisp on the outside and soft when pierced with a sharp knife. Remove from the oven and leave to cool. Place the beet leaves in a large serving bowl, along with the mixed salad leaves. When they are cool enough to handle, slice the beets into halves or quarters and add to the salad, along with the tarragon leaves, avocado, and chicken. In a suitable container, mix together the ingredients for the dressing. Drizzle the vinegar dressing over the salad and toss it lightly. Season with lots of freshly ground black pepper and a little sea salt. Serve immediately.

## PENNE WITH WATERCRESS PESTO (SERVES 1)

*Other than being thrown into a salad, watercress is often overlooked. So here's a great way to work this iron-rich vegetable into your diet: Use it to make some fresh pesto. This recipe makes enough pesto so that you'll have some left to refrigerate for another day.*

2 1/2 cups watercress, washed and dried

1 garlic clove, crushed

3 1/4 cups pine nuts, toasted, plus extra
  for serving

4 Tbs. freshly grated Parmesan cheese, plus
  extra for serving

2 Tbs. olive oil

5/8 cup dried penne

To make the pesto, place all the ingredients except the pasta into a food processor, and process into a smooth paste. Season with some freshly ground black pepper and a little sea salt. Meanwhile, bring a pan of salted water to the boil, drop in the penne, and cook according to the package instructions. Drain the penne, leaving about 4 Tbs. of the cooking liquid in the pan. Stir in 4 Tbs. of the watercress pesto and toss. Spoon the pesto-coated penne into a warmed pasta bowl; sprinkle with some Parmesan shavings and maybe a few toasted pine nuts.

# cut down on caffeine and savor the flavor

Coffee- and tea-drinking habits vary from individual to individual, as do the effects these beverages can have. Some people feel stimulated after drinking coffee or tea, while others feel wired, anxious, headachy, and dehydrated, and as if that weren't enough, their moods and energy levels swing all over the place, too.

From a nutritional perspective, less is more when it comes to coffee and tea. Overconsumption of caffeine reduces the body's ability to absorb such minerals as iron (disastrous if you have iron-deficiency anemia or heavy periods) and increases the loss of calcium from the bones. While a cup of fresh coffee can kick-start a lazy gut and relieve constipation, it may equally aggravate an irritated, acidic digestive system—the last thing you need if you're already feeling anxious.

## caffeine contents

I find a double espresso a good compromise because it doesn't contain as much caffeine (45–100mg) as filter, percolated, or French press coffee (60–120mg); it doesn't make me feel jittery, but still acts as a stimulant. The reason for espresso's low caffeine content is the speed with which the steam is blasted through the coffee beans, which means that little caffeine ends up in the cup. Instant coffees, which are made from dried infusions that have been spray- or freeze-dried, contain slightly less caffeine (70mg) than fresh coffee. Their downside, however, is their inferior taste, while percolated and French press coffee have been shown to increase levels of "bad" cholesterol (LPL). You may find that adding milk slows down the caffeine "hit" of a cup of coffee. If you use soy or oat milk, it is usually best to let the coffee cool slightly before adding, as it can curdle.

## hot and healing

Among coffee's and tea's plus points are the antioxidants they contain, which fend off heart disease, delay the aging process, and speed recovery from a cold or infection. Even decaffeinated products pack a powerful antioxidant punch; look for labels that indicate caffeine has been removed by the water method. If you don't find this description on the label, assume that the product's been exposed to unhealthful chemicals. Research also supports the theory that caffeine can help in allaying the symptoms of Alzheimer's.

To keep tea leaves and tea bags fresher for longer, store them, along with ground coffee, in dark, airtight containers in a cool cabinet, away from strong-smelling items like garlic and spices. Alternatively, you might keep ground coffee in the refrigerator and coffee beans in the freezer. A package of ground coffee should be consumed within three to four weeks of opening.

## the case for tea

Tea contains less caffeine (40mg) than coffee, which makes its effect on the body gentler; and when you consider that tea, like coffee, contains antioxidants, there's a lot to be said for it. However tea is packed with tannins, which can irritate sensitive digestive systems and cause constipation.

## the perfect cup of tea

First, warm your best china teapot by filling it with hot water. Tip the hot water away, then pop your chosen tea leaves into the pot. Fill your kettle with freshly drawn water. Boil the kettle, fill your teapot, and leave the tea leaves to infuse for 3–4 minutes, according to taste.

There's a wide variety of teas to choose from, including black and green tea, Darjeeling, Assam, Earl Grey, and lapsang souchong, to name but a few. Although exceedingly expensive, white tea, the most delicate of all, offers the richest concentration of antioxidants, which makes it a great anti-aging aid. If you're interested in harnessing the antioxidant qualities of white tea, some of the varieties available include white peony, white Darjeeling, and snowbud. In the summer, iced teas are wonderfully refreshing. Here's how to make two of my favorites.

## COOL AND SWEET (SERVES 1)

Make a fresh pot of tea with your favorite leaves. When it has brewed, strain it into a cocktail shaker. Add 1 tsp. brown sugar and a generous dash of fresh lemon juice. Chill the shaker. Place a few ice cubes in the bottom of some large highball glasses, shake the shaker vigorously, and then pour the tea into the glasses. Garnish with slices of lemon and serve with straws.

## CHILLED AND ZINGY (SERVES 1)

Place some ice in a cocktail shaker, pour in 1 cup freshly brewed, cooled black tea, such as English breakfast tea, and then add a dash of orange syrup and another of freshly squeezed lemon juice. Place 4 ice cubes in a 12-oz. glass, shake the cocktail shaker vigorously, and then strain the tea into the glass. Garnish with slices of lemon and orange with the peel removed.

# keep a clear head by limiting your alcohol intake

Many of us like to drink alcohol, and there's no reason why you shouldn't, as long as you resist the temptation to overindulge. The cultural tide is moving away from lunchtime drinking, which affects our bodies particularly badly, and people are increasingly more likely to enjoy a glass of wine with a meal than they are to indulge in several cocktails after work. Compared to many countries, alcohol consumption in the United States is quite low; in a list of countries ranked according to per capita consumption of alcohol, the U.S. ranked only 26th. However, surveys have shown that over 13 percent of adults in this country succumb to alcohol abuse or dependence (that is, alcoholism) at some point in their lives. Indeed, some people would argue that the legislation targeting cannabis would be better applied to alcohol, which, they say, is far more damaging to our health, both as individuals and as a society. Hmmm: a drug and an intoxicant it may be, yet alcohol needn't be harmful.

Let's look at alcohol's downsides. An intake of more than 3 drinks a day for men and 2 drinks for women is thought to increase the risk of developing hypertension and obesity, raising the specter of heart disease. (The reason for the difference in the recommended limits is that women have both smaller livers and less of the alcohol-protecting enzyme ADH than men and therefore don't metabolize alcohol as efficiently.) It may also increase your chances of developing osteoporosis and certain cancers, of suffering damage to your liver and pancreas, and of exacerbating depression and suppressing energy levels on a day-to-day basis.

## to your good health

Red wine, it seems, contains enough flavonoids to protect us from some of the free-radical damage that causes cirrhosis and pancreatitis (diseases that kill many alcoholics), also warding off heart disease and cancer. In addition, red wine's flavonoids have anti-aging properties (and may even help to fend off the onset of Alzheimer's) and the power to discourage cholesterol and other blood fats from oxidizing and to increase levels of "good" cholesterol (HDL). If you have diabetes, further benefits are the prevention of blindness and of kidney and circulation problems.

Some wines contain more flavonoids than others. Darker, tannin-packed red wines generally offer the most, so Chianti, Cabernet Sauvignon, and Merlot lead the way, with Pinot Noir and Rioja following on their heels, and Beaujolais, Côtes du Rhône, and white and rosé wines bringing up the rear. If you're teetotal or don't like red wine, an alternative is red grape juice; but because it's exposed to the air during production, some of the valuable flavonoids are lost.

Although a moderate consumption of alcohol containing antioxidant flavonoids is thought to have a protective effect, there comes a point at which the benefits are outweighed by the dangers of overconsumption. All in all, it's safer to glean your antioxidants from food. Yet heavy drinkers tend to have both a poor diet and a reduced capacity for absorbing nutrients, a double whammy that may result in deficiencies of vitamins B1 and B6, beta carotene, folate, vitamin C, and zinc. While beer contains some B vitamins, and red wine contains iron, the disadvantages of heavy drinking overshadow this.

So make no mistake: having more than 2 drinks a day is bad news, not least because really heavy drinking ages the kidneys, heart, and brain and speeds up other aspects of the aging process. Stick to 2 drinks a day or fewer, however, and you'll be encouraging your blood platelets to become less sticky, reducing the risk of having a heart attack.

## healthy measures

What does this all mean in practice? Well, it's better to drink small amounts of your designated maximum regularly—a couple of glasses five days a week—than to consume the whole amount in one binge-drinking session. What counts as a "drink"? For wine, a "drink" is 5 ounces (just under one-fifth of a bottle); for beer, it's 12 ounces; for 80-proof whiskey and comparable spirits, it's 1½ ounces. Ideally aim for a couple of alcohol-free days a week to allow your body to recover. Not drinking during the week, but savoring a few glasses at the weekend works for me. You may have found that only a couple of drinks at the end of a tiring day disrupts your sleeping patterns, so that you feel devoid of energy the next day. If you're short, small-framed, or overweight, be warned that alcohol's negative effects can hit you really hard.

The guidelines regarding drinking alcohol during pregnancy are rather controversial. Although some experts say that having 1 or 2 drinks once or twice a week is fine, I'm inclined to agree with the research that shows regularly drinking even small amounts isn't good for your unborn baby. And because alcohol reduces your chances of hitting the baby jackpot, I'd advocate drastically limiting your alcohol consumption if you're trying to conceive.

Whatever your sex, drink only when you have food in your stomach to cushion alcohol's negative effects—energy crashes and plummeting blood-sugar levels that give a false appetite, as well as the aggravation of digestive problems like indigestion, hiatus hernia, and ulcers. Drink on an empty stomach and you'll feel totally washed out at best—particularly if you're already tired and stressed—and will be lucky if you don't wake up the next morning with a crippling hangover (see pages 82–3). But hold on—wasn't the whole point of drinking last night an attempt to feel good?

# increase your strength
# with body-boosting protein

Protein is vital if the body is to build strong muscles, repair tissues, and maintain effective immune and hormonal systems. Once you've eaten a protein-rich food, it is broken down by digestive enzymes and absorbed into the blood as amino acids, which the body uses to build and repair cells or fuel spurts of energy, storing any extra as fat. There are two types of amino acid: essential and non-essential. Although the body can generate non-essential amino acids from non-dietary sources, it can obtain essential amino acids only from food, which is why you need to make sure that your daily diet contains an adequate supply of them.

Meat, poultry, game, fish and shellfish, eggs, dairy, and soy products (like soy milk, yogurt, and tofu) contain all the essential amino acids. Beans and other legumes, grains, nuts, seeds, and manufactured vegetable-protein foods contain protein, but not all the essential amino acids. They can, however, be combined (legumes with grains or nuts, for example) to give the body its daily protein requirement.

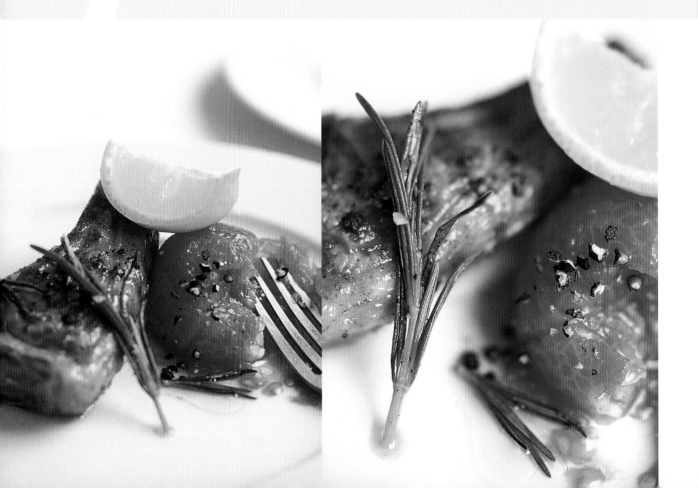

## the dangers of high-protein diets

There's a lot of controversy about the amount of protein that our bodies need, perhaps because going on high-protein, low-carbohydrate diets has trimmed down many celebrities. And while a high-protein diet seems to help people to lose weight and feel more energized, unlike a diet that is loaded with starchy carbohydrates, there are dangers associated with going down this path.

A person weighing 130 lb. (59 kg) needs only a little more than 1½ oz. of protein a day. The problem with extreme diets that advocate eating primarily protein with very little else—and certainly hardly any carbohydrates—is that not only can the protein that is surplus to the body's immediate requirements be stored as fat (particularly if it is animal protein), but it increases calcium loss from the bones, raising the specter of osteoporosis and also adversely affecting kidney function and sometimes blood pressure. And if you consume less than the 4 oz. of carbohydrates that your body requires a day, it is likely to enter a state called ketosis, which makes your mouth taste metallic and your concentration lapse.

## achieving a balance

I'd advise you to have a piece of lean protein about the size of a chicken breast for your main meal, plus a portion half this size in a smaller meal or snack. Try my Broiled Lamb Chops with Crushed Tomatoes (see page 33) for a speedy weekday dinner or my Sage Roast Pork for a relaxed weekend dinner (see page 32). It's best to opt for lean meat rather than fatty or cured meats or meat products, such as sausages and salamis, in order to reduce your saturated-fat and salt intakes. Oily fish (including salmon, fresh tuna, mackerel, and sardines) not only are great sources of protein but also contain the omega-3 fatty acids, which offer numerous benefits to health. If you want to eat more protein than this guideline, lean toward such non-animal proteins as legumes, soy, and nuts (see pages 30–31). Nuts, seeds, and vegetable oils are rich in omega-6 fatty acids, which also reduce the risk of heart disease.

In fact, it's easy to follow a compromise: a protein-and-carbohydrate diet that encourages you to lose weight and feel energetic while also protecting your bones and metabolism. One suggestion is to have a meal that contains a high-fiber carbohydrate, perhaps a couple of slices of whole-wheat toast or my Cardamom Rice Milk Porridge (see page 42) for breakfast, and then to base the rest of the day around protein-rich foods, fruits, vegetables, and legumes. Alternatively, enjoying a carbohydrate-rich meal at the end of the day—maybe a plate of risotto or pasta—will make you feel relaxed and sleepy. Try my soothing Mushroom Risotto (see page 136).

## can vegetarians take the pace of a busy lifestyle?

Vegetarians can certainly lead as active lives as meat eaters, although there's a greater danger that they may deprive their bodies of such essential nutrients as protein, vitamin $B_{12}$, iron, calcium, and zinc. This is why it's vital that vegetarians both understand the body's nutritional requirements and eat plenty of the foods that will fulfill them. The main vegetarian sources of protein are

- Soy and its products
- Legumes, including beans, chickpeas, and lentils (fresh, dried, or canned)
- Grains, such as whole-wheat bread and oats
- Dairy foods, such as yogurt, cheese, and milk

In terms of quantity, vegetarians should aim to eat one full portion of a protein-packed food as a main meal and half a portion in a smaller meal: a portion equates to 1 scant cup legumes (cooked weight), 1 generous 3/4 cup nuts, 8 oz. tofu or a couple of eggs. If you eat a single serving of my Worth-the-effort Baked Beans (see page 33) or my Fresh Borlotti Beans with Thyme (see page 22), then you'll reach your daily protein target in one meal.

## fortify your diet

Although most vegetarian foods are packed with vitamins and minerals, they lack $B_{12}$, a vitamin that maintains the health of the blood and nervous system, and a sustained lack of which can cause anemia and irreversible nerve damage. To avert these dangers, make sure that your diet includes either vitamin $B_{12}$-rich eggs and dairy foods or, if you're a vegan, foods that have been fortified with $B_{12}$, such as soy products and some breakfast cereals.

## iron providers

Another potential pitfall for busy vegetarians is a deficiency in iron, which the body requires to manufacture the hemoglobin in red blood cells, and a lack of which can cause anemia. The following non-animal foods are relatively rich in iron:

- Granola and whole-wheat bread
- Dark green, leafy vegetables, particularly spinach
- Beans and lentils
- Nuts and seeds, especially pistachios, cashews, sesame seeds, and pine nuts
- Oatmeal
- Dried fruit, particularly figs and apricots
- Eggs

Eat as many of these iron providers as you can, and help your body to glean as much of this essential nutrient as possible by teaming them with a food that contains vitamin C—orange juice, citrus and kiwi fruits, and berries, for instance—which encourages the gut to absorb iron, and by limiting your intake of caffeine-containing drinks, which hinder the body's absorption of iron.

Finally, dairy foods are the best sources of calcium (see pages 36–7), but if you're a vegan, eat plenty of dark green, leafy vegetables (like curly kale, spinach, and watercress), seeds (particularly tahini made from sesame seeds, sunflower seeds, and linseeds), nuts (especially almonds and brazil nuts), dried fruit, and tofu. These foods will also boost your levels of zinc, a nutrient that is required to keep your immune system and libido healthy.

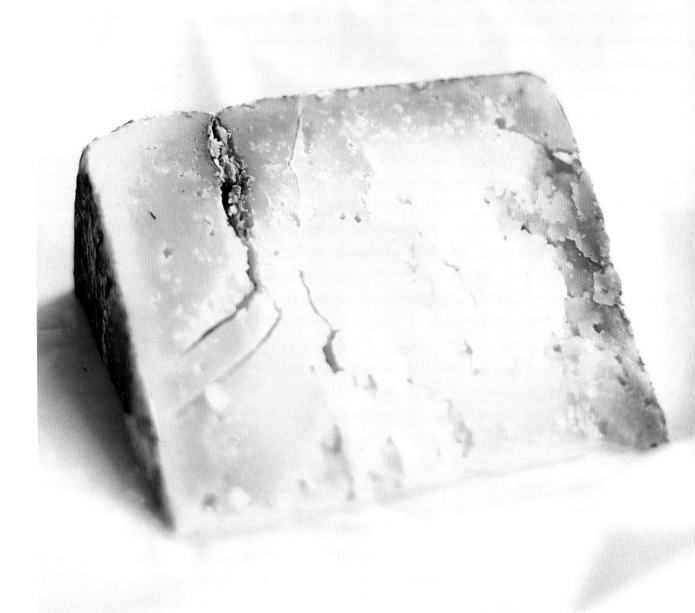

## SAGE ROAST PORK (SERVES 6)

*Pork is coming back into fashion. I love it both hot, with plenty of steamed vegetables, and cold, sandwiched between slices of whole-wheat bread with a little mayonnaise and applesauce—two good standbys to have in your fridge. If possible, ask a butcher to prepare a crown roast, cutting the meat almost away from the bone and breaking the bones to make carving easier.*

| | |
|---|---|
| 3$1/4$ lbs. loin of pork, with rib bones, trimmed | 2 sprigs of fresh sage |
| 6 garlic cloves, crushed | 3 Tbs. olive oil |

Heat the oven to 400°. Using a sharp knife, make several incisions all the way around the loin. Make a paste (you could do this in a food processor) with the rest of the ingredients and season with some freshly ground black pepper and a little sea salt. Press a small amount of the paste into each incision, and then rub the rest all over the surface of the meat (including where it was attached to the bone). Reattach the meat to the bone with string or skewers, and then transfer to a roasting pan. Bake in the oven for 1$1/2$ hours, or until it is done to your taste, basting frequently with the melted fat that has collected in the bottom of the roasting pan.

## BEAN AND HAZELNUT LOAF (SERVES 3–4)

*An easy protein-rich loaf that will last a few days. It can be used in sandwiches or served with vegetables or salad.*

| | |
|---|---|
| 2 large portobello mushrooms, thickly sliced | 1/8 cup hazelnuts, chopped |
| 2 Tbs. olive oil | 2 oz. sharp cheddar cheese, grated |
| generous 1/2 cup black-eyed peas, drained | 1/2 tsp. Dijon mustard |
| generous 1/2 cup chickpeas, drained | 1 Tbs. chopped cilantro |
| 2 shallots, finely chopped | 1 Tbs. fresh chopped parsley |
| 1 green onion, thinly sliced | 2 organic eggs |
| 2 small leeks, cleaned and finely sliced | dash of tamari |
| 2 garlic cloves, crushed | dash of Tabasco sauce |

Heat the oven to 375°. Sauté the mushrooms in a little olive oil. Place the mushrooms with all the other ingredients in a blender and blend lightly until combined but still crunchy in texture. Season to taste with some freshly ground black pepper and a little sea salt. Now transfer the mixture to a bread pan, lined with waxed paper, and bake it in the oven for approximately 40 minutes, or until the loaf is set and golden brown on top. Either serve the loaf at once or keep it in the fridge to enjoy cold with salads or in sandwiches, or to heat up in the microwave whenever you want some.

## BROILED LAMB CHOPS WITH CRUSHED TOMATOES (SERVES 4)

*For the marinade*

3 Tbs. olive oil

juice of 1/2 lemon (or more to taste)

2 garlic cloves, crushed

1 sprig of fresh rosemary

4 lamb chops

4 tomatoes

1 lemon, cut into quarters, for serving

Combine all the ingredients for the marinade with some freshly ground black pepper. Marinate the lamb for about 1 hour. Meanwhile, take a bath or read to relax and unwind. Heat the broiler to a high temperature. Sprinkle the chops with sea salt, and cook them under the hot broiler for 10–15 minutes, turning once, until they are well browned but still pink and juicy inside. While the chops are cooking, also heat the tomatoes under the broiler until they become soft enough to enable you to peel off the skin easily. Transfer the chops to the plates; place 1 lemon quarter on each and 1 tomato to the side. Crush the tomatoes with a fork before serving.

## WORTH-THE-EFFORT BAKED BEANS (SERVES 6)

*I'm a huge baked bean fan. I grab them out of a can if I'm pushed, but at weekends I'll take the time to make my own, as they freeze well and can be defrosted in minutes. They're also good for an informal supper with friends, served with crusty bread and red wine.*

1 1/8 lbs. 2oz small white cannellini beans, soaked overnight in cold water

2 sprigs of fresh sage

3/8 cup olive oil

2 garlic cloves, crushed

5 ripe tomatoes, skinned and chopped

Drain the beans, which have been soaked overnight, place them in a saucepan with enough fresh water to cover them, and add 1 of the sprigs of fresh sage and 2 Tbs. of the olive oil. Bring the water to the boil, and then simmer for about 1 1/2 hours, or until the beans are tender, adding a little sea salt when they begin to soften. Remove the beans from the pan and drain them. Gently heat (but do not fry) the remaining olive oil with the garlic and the remaining sage, over a low flame, to infuse the oil with the aromatic flavors. Add the tomatoes and simmer for 10 minutes. Now add the drained beans, season with some freshly ground black pepper and a little sea salt, and cook for another 5 minutes or so. You should end up with a generous amount of sauce.

# choose full-fat foods for full flavor

The low-fat lifestyle isn't healthy! Yes, you read it right: not only have I seen this myself in patient after patient, but after decades of warning us about the myriad evils of full-fat foods, nutritional authorities on both sides of the Atlantic are starting to backtrack and admit that the conventional advice may be flawed.

As you may have experienced, switching to low-fat products when trying to lose weight rarely works, because they simply don't make you feel full; so, minutes after eating, you're scouting around for something else to satisfy your stomach. You may tell yourself that because such foods are low in fat it's okay to eat double the amount. You'd be wrong: they may contain less fat than their high-fat counterparts, but like many carbohydrates, they are loaded with more sugar, which sends your body's production of insulin into overdrive and will ultimately cause you to pile on the pounds, not shed them.

## the low-fat myth

In terms of taste, as well as nutritional content, low-fat foods are poor substitutes. Their lack of flavor is important: because the taste buds aren't stimulated, they, in turn, fail to tell the hypothalamus—the part of the brain that tells you when you're satisfied—that it's time to stop eating. Full-fat foods, on the other hand, register more swiftly with both the taste buds and the hypothalamus, meaning you'll feel fuller faster, and having eaten less. It's also vital that the body receive some fat, and not just because fat injects a concentrated source of energy. Besides providing the fuel that enables the body to metabolize hormones (particularly sex hormones) and repair tissues, fat contains the fat-soluble vitamins A, D, E, and K, all of which are essential for health, and a lack of which may cause defects in unborn babies. And by plumping the skin up, subcutaneous fat also makes the skin smooth and pliable.

## I'm confused: Can I binge on French fries?

I'm not a fan of low-fat products, but I'm not advocating stuffing yourself with deep-fried foods, either. The key to enjoying all of the benefits of fat, but none of its disadvantages, is to give your body the correct type and ensure that it makes up 30–35 percent of your daily consumption. There are two main types: saturated fat (animal products like meat and full-fat dairy foods) and unsaturated fat (vegetable products like cooking oils, avocados, nuts and seeds, and also oily fish). If you overindulge in saturated fats, including fried foods, you run the risk of raising your cholesterol level, clogging up your arteries and ultimately developing heart disease; enjoy unsaturated fats in moderation, and you'll be nurturing, not harming, your body, so it is these that you should focus on eating.

## vegetable oils and omega oils

The unsaturated-fat family tree branches into monounsaturated, polyunsaturated, and hydrogenated fats. Of these, such monounsaturated fats as olive oil are the healthiest. Polyunsaturated and hydrogenated fats—margarines, low-fat, and olive-based spreads—are, however, best treated with caution, because many contain trans fatty acids, which have been linked with the development of heart disease and cancer through their encouragement of free-radical activity within the body.

Besides using vegetable oils (olive oil is the most healthful, followed by safflower and sunflower oil) when cooking and dressing salads, supply your body with a regular dose of beneficial omega oils by eating more oily fish, including fresh tuna (not canned), wild salmon (rather than farmed), herrings, trout, and mackerel. Also known as omega-3 and omega-6 fatty acids, omega oils have been shown to ward off heart disease and certain cancers, as well as alleviate some skin conditions. Not only that, but they are rich in protein and taste delicious!

I also like to use hempseed oil—the oil with the perfect omega-3 and omega-6 fatty acid balance—in salad dressings. Sadly, you can't cook with hemp oil, but try half hemp oil and half olive oil in a dressing for a good balance of health versus taste.

## putting the theory into practice

- You can still titillate your taste buds by enjoying saturated fats, but only a little, so regard whole milk, cheese, yogurt, cream, and butter as occasional treats.
- Wean yourself off deep-fried fast foods and instead learn to love the classic Mediterranean diet, which revolves around lots of olive oil, oily fish, and vegetables.
- Eat oily fish three times a week, but reduce your meat consumption. When shopping for red meat, choose lean cuts over fatty, and try to buy organic, free-range meat, which contains less saturated fat than farmed meat and game.
- Use a spoonful of oil high in monounsaturates, such as olive, walnut, or sunflower oil, for frying instead of butter. Never overheat cooking oil (if it's smoking in the pan, it's too hot) or reuse it, as this will produce harmful trans fatty acids.
- Cut down on polyunsaturated vegetable oils and spreads, along with foods that contain hydrogenated vegetable oils or fats.
- To preserve their taste and shelf life, store monounsaturated oils in dark glass bottles in the fridge.
- Transform regular olive oil into an aromatic herbal oil by adding your favorite chopped fresh herbs— perhaps rosemary, thyme, sage, or oregano—to the bottle. Not only will the infused oil taste great, but herbs have numerous beneficial properties (thyme, for example, provides brain-boosting antioxidants), as do cloves, nutmeg, and pepper. Some of the best olive oils have an amazingly stimulating pepper kick.

# nurture your body with precious minerals

We often focus on vitamins, but it's essential to consider minerals, too—in particular, calcium, magnesium, zinc, and iron. It's important to include plenty of dairy products in your diet because of their high calcium and vitamin D content, nutrients that help to build strong bones and thus reduce the risk of developing osteoporosis, or brittle-bone disease (the commonest cause of disability after fifty, especially in women).

Osteoporosis sufferers are often unaware of their condition until they experience their first fracture in later life. It is preventable, if you eat to beat it from childhood. Bone mass, which consists of calcium, builds during our early years, our bones becoming harder until, by our late teens, the long bones in the arms and legs have reached their maximum strength and length. After twenty, our bones lose density, a decline that accelerates in postmenopausal women. The more bone mass you accumulate as a child and young adult, the greater the cushion against developing osteoporosis when you pass thirty, when new bone tissue is no longer deposited.

Children must eat a plentiful supply of calcium, but adults should consume 2½ cups milk and 4½ oz. cheese or a large tub of yogurt each day. Meet this target with a yogurt smoothie for breakfast, cheese in a sandwich for lunch or sprinkled over pasta for supper, with a glass of milk at bedtime. If you can't tolerate cow's milk, think about calcium-enriched soy milk. Goat's, sheep's, oat, and rice milks are other options, although lactose-intolerant people should lean toward soy, oat, and rice milks and their products.

## maximize calcium absorption

Vitamin D is important, since it assists your body in absorbing calcium from the gut; regular exposure to the sun's ultraviolet rays triggers the skin's production of this nutrient. Spend some time outside every day, especially during the summer months, to build up your body's vitamin D reserves—just don't forget the sunscreen! (There is also evidence to show that high levels of vitamin D within the body can prevent certain cancers from striking—notably cancer of the breast, ovary, womb, prostate gland, esophagus, stomach, colon, and rectum—through vitamin D's ability to inhibit the development and spread of malignant tumors.) Failing that, and especially in winter, good nutritional alternatives include, conveniently enough, dairy products and oily fish. Remember, both you and your children can further strengthen your bones by staying as active as possible.

Besides warding off osteoporosis, a diet that contains high levels of calcium is important for the healthy functioning of the heart, muscles, and nerves, having been shown to reduce the incidence of heart disease and to lower high blood pressure (see pages 122–5). A calcium-rich diet, in tandem with a high vitamin D intake, is essential in improving the gut's ability to absorb this nutrient, and hence its transformation into healthy bone mass. There's an array of calcium-packed foods to choose from: along with dairy products like yogurt, milk and cheese (particularly Parmesan, Gruyère, cheddar, and mozzarella), the list includes canned salmon, sardines, tofu, and fortified soy milk, beans (such as baked beans), chickpeas, leafy green vegetables, broccoli, almonds, dried figs, granola, white bread, dried seaweed, and milk chocolate.

To provide your body with vitamin D, focus on oily fish like sardines, mackerel, fresh tuna, and salmon, cod-liver oil, eggs, margarine, butter, milk, and yogurt. The omega-3 and 6 fatty acids that oily fish also contain (as do seeds, evening primrose, starflower, and borage oils) encourage the gut to absorb calcium, too, making it well worth either boosting your intake of oily fish or, if that doesn't appeal, taking a supplement of omega oil (or of any of the aforementioned herbal oils). And besides offering other benefits to health, omega oils both reduce calcium wastage within the body and direct that which the body does absorb straight to the bones. An additional helpful nutrient is vitamin K, which not only is essential for bone growth and repair, but also is a promoter of calcium absorption. It is generated by bifido bacteria within the gut, so establish a thriving colony of "good" bacteria by either eating live, probiotic yogurt or taking a supplement.

## watch your fiber intake

If boosting your calcium is a priority—maybe you're pregnant or advanced in years—be warned that eating foods that are high in insoluble fiber (such as bran-packed cereals, granola and whole-wheat bread) with a source of calcium (a cheese sandwich made with whole-wheat bread, for example) can decrease the body's absorption of calcium, due to the blocking action of the fiber's phytates. The oxalates in rhubarb, spinach, beets and chard, as well as the tannins in coffee and tea, have a similar inhibiting effect, although you can get around the tannin problem by allowing some time between a calcium-rich meal and a cup of tea or coffee (for instance, having a cup of tea mid-morning, rather than an espresso directly after lunch).

All of these nutritional strategies are far preferable to taking large doses of calcium in the form of supplements, which can hinder the body's absorption of iron and consequently increase your vulnerability to iron-deficiency anemia. So, don't be tempted to cheat!

## don't forget magnesium, zinc, and iron

A high magnesium intake has been linked with the alleviation of premenstrual syndrome, a lower incidence of heart disease, and an improvement in lung function in asthmatics. If you are deficient in magnesium, your body will feel weak, particularly your muscles, which may have a tendency to cramp at night; you may lose your appetite, and with it your energy; and if you have insufficient levels of magnesium in your blood, your body will draw it from your bones, increasing your risk of developing osteoporosis. If you are diabetic, low magnesium levels can cause increased resistance to insulin and other complications. The best sources of magnesium are nuts, particularly brazil nuts, pine nuts, seeds, soy beans, and tofu, along with licorice and cocoa powder. Iron-rich foods include dark green, leafy vegetables, legumes, dried fruits, whole grains, eggs, cashew nuts, lean red meat, and variety meats.

## supplementary benefits?

There may be occasions when time and willpower are in such short supply that you're tempted to take a supplement to cover all the nutritional bases. Although this may seem logical, it's unwise, for two main reasons. Firstly, it can be a waste of your hard-earned cash, as you'll be swallowing nutrients that your body doesn't need; you'll literally be flushing them away. Secondly, bombarding your body with vitamin and mineral supplements can cause a nutritional imbalance. Some nutrients even hinder the absorption of other essentials. More is not always better. Supplements can even be harmful.

If you still believe that supplements may be the answer for you, see a state-registered dietitian (member of ADA), who will assess your individual needs impartially, without being under financial pressure to sell you supplements (which can be a problem in health-food stores). A dietition will also make sure that you won't be at risk of toxicity and that your symptoms aren't due to an underlying medical condition that needs specific treatment (just two of the reasons why self-diagnosis and prescription are very inadvisable).

Although there are rare instances when fortified, functional foods that provide extra nutrients can be useful (such as kids' snacks and drinks with added calcium), these products are not only expensive but also usually highly processed, full of sugar, fat, salt, or additives, and generally not that healthful. They may appear to offer a shortcut to health, but seldom do. It's far better to stick to incorporating as many simple, unprocessed, nutrient-rich foods as possible into your diet.

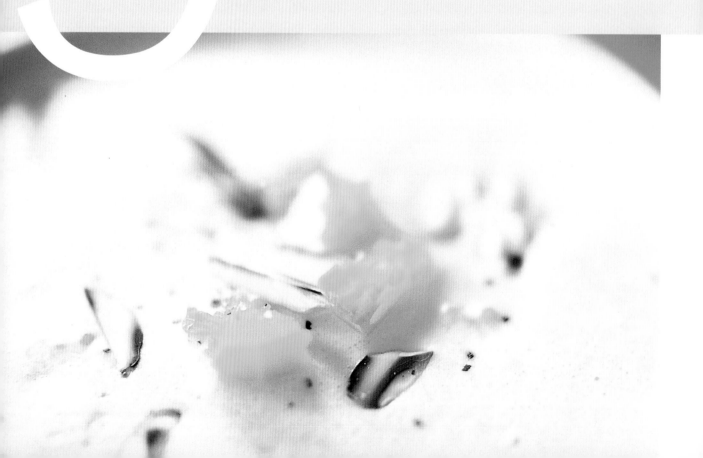

## RASPBERRY AND BANANA SOY SHAKE (SERVES 1)

*Calcium-enriched soy is a great way to boost your calcium intake, especially if you can't tolerate dairy products. For me, this is a good way to start a draining day, with something substantial, but not heavy on the stomach. There is no comparison between the flavor of a homemade fruit shake and the bought variety. Simply add whatever fruits you have available—although raspberries and bananas make such a perfect combination that they are worth buying specially—to some soy yogurt for a melt-in-the-mouth experience for one.*

Place 5/8 cup fresh raspberries and 1 roughly chopped banana in a blender or food processor and blend until smooth. Add 3/4 cup calcium-enriched soya yogurt and blend again, until the ingredients have been thoroughly mixed. Stir in some clear honey to taste. Now sieve the mixture into a bowl, drop a little ice into a glass, pour in the shake, and savor at once.

## PUMPKIN SOUP WITH ALMONDS (SERVES 4)

*Milk and almonds are usually combined in sweet foods, but here is a way to get a savory calcium hit, which is also a comforting de-stressing soup.*

| | |
|---|---|
| **4 cups pumpkin flesh, skinned, deseeded, and diced** | **freshly grated nutmeg** |
| | **1 1/4 cups light cream** |
| **3 3/4 cups milk** | **4 Tbs. chopped, toasted almonds** |

Place the pumpkin in a saucepan with the milk and the nutmeg to taste. Season with some freshly ground black pepper and a little sea salt. Bring to the boil and simmer for about 30 minutes, or until the pumpkin is tender. Pour the soup into a blender, and process it until smooth. Then return it to the saucepan and stir in the cream. Divide among four soup plates and sprinkle 1 Tbs. almonds over each before serving.

## HONEY ICE CREAM (SERVES 4–6)

*It's worth investing in a self-refrigerating ice-cream maker, which, although not cheap, can make this scented-honey ice cream and other delicious desserts in literally minutes. I also use mine to make Nigel Slater's Chocolate Ice Cream (see page 75).*

Break 1 egg into a bowl, and add 4 egg yolks and 1/3 cup (scant) scented honey (acacia, for example). Set the bowl over a saucepan containing boiling water, and beat until the mixture becomes thick and pale. In a separate bowl, beat 1 1/4 cups heavy cream until it is stiff, then fold it into the egg mixture. Pour into the ice-cream maker and follow the instructions until the ice cream is frozen.

# eat whole grains for a healthy balanced body

Ever since Dr. Kellogg launched his high-fiber breakfast cereals, over a century ago, we've been told that eating some high-fiber food every day is good for us. This is why we're encouraged to eat such whole grains as whole-wheat bread and brown rice in preference to their refined counterparts. While most of us know that whole-grain foods promote regular action in the bowel department, their protective effect against conditions such as heart disease, cancer, and diabetes may come as news to you.

Grains such as wheat and rice are made up of a soft, inner part (the endosperm) and two fibrous, outer parts (the germ and bran). During refining, the germ and bran are lost, and with them a good proportion of the grain's fiber content, so that when the grain is eaten, the rate at which it releases sugar into the bloodstream is speeded up. The problem is, the more rapidly sugar is absorbed into the bloodstream, the more insulin the pancreas secretes to compensate. One of insulin's effects is to stimulate the production of cholesterol, which means that an overproduction of insulin can result not only in diabetes but also in heart disease. Another negative effect of the refining process is that it deprives the grain of vital nutrients, including folic acid, vitamins E, B1, B5, and B6 and the minerals iron, zinc, magnesium, selenium, and copper, some of which ward off heart disease and others cancer.

Besides releasing energy slowly into the body, keeping us fuller for longer, whole grains therefore offer significant nutritional advantages over their refined versions. This is backed up by the statistics: studies have shown that eating plenty of whole grains cuts the danger of developing diabetes by half and reduces the likelihood of succumbing to heart disease by a third, while having four servings of whole-grain foods a week may lower the cancer risk by 40 percent.

## friendly fibers

Certain fibers can fend off food poisoning, bowel conditions, and liver cancer, too. Called oligosaccharides, these soluble, prebiotic fibers promote the growth of "good" bifido bacteria in the gut by providing them with a food source. And when there are teeming levels of bifido bacteria in the gut, the "bad" disease-causing bacteria find themselves fighting a battle for survival. A gut that contains healthy levels of bifido bacteria is also better able to absorb minerals, while other benefits include the blood-sugar-regulating acids that they generate and their apparent ability both to discourage the body from laying down fat stores and to boost the immune system.

I'd therefore recommend eating plenty of prebiotic foods, including all fruits and vegetables, but especially artichokes, onions, leeks, oats, Belgian endive, wheat, and bananas. Bear in mind. though, that their prebiotic values degrade over time, so try to eat these foods as soon as possible after buying them. And because antibiotics don't distinguish between "good" and "bad" bacteria and target them all, if you've been prescribed these drugs, I'd advise taking a daily 5–10g prebiotic supplement for a couple of weeks after you've finished the course.

Another way of nurturing a healthy bacterial balance, particularly after you've had a stomach upset, is either to eat live, ideally organic, yogurt, which contains "good" probiotic bacteria like lactobacillus, acidophilus, and bifidus, or to take probiotic supplements, such as acidophilus capsules. Exposure to heat and light will kill these benevolent bacteria, so make sure that you buy refrigerated yogurts and supplements, and store them in the fridge.

## fiber tips

- Buy whole-wheat bread (brown bread is often white bread that has been dyed and contains no more fiber).
- Incorporate prebiotic foods, such as artichokes, onions, and leeks, into your diet gradually, as they may initially cause bloating.
- Start the day with fresh fruit, perhaps sliced over your breakfast cereal or blended with probiotic yogurt to make a smoothie, or have oatmeal or granola.
- Out of sight is out of mind, so place fruit in a prominent position at home or on your desk.
- Snack on dried fruits, but only a few at a time. Try mixing dried and fresh fruits—Medjool dates with banana slices, for example. Buy dried fruits that haven't been exposed to sulfur dioxide ($SO_2$).
- Keep a supply of whole-wheat crisp breads handy to team with salads and soups for lunch. Also stock up on whole-grain cookies, which make ideal after-work snacks; and see My Favorite Oatcakes on page 80.
- Include lots of canned or dried (soaked) legumes in your diet: add canned legumes to ready-made soups or buy soups based on lentils and beans; indulge yourself with baked beans on toast (see my Worth-the-effort Baked Beans on page 33); add lentils to casseroles or serve them instead of potatoes, and try your hand at making dhal.
- Buy whole-grain rice and pasta, instead of their refined counterparts.
- Leave the skins on baked potatoes. Although microwaving saves time, if a crisp-skinned, fluffy-centered baked potato is what you desire, rub some olive oil over the skin, place it in a hot oven, and then relax while it's baking.
- Drink at least 5 pints of water over the course of each day to aid your digestion. Sip one glass every hour to stagger your intake and enable your kidneys to process it better (see pages 12–13).

## BRAN FLAKES WITH TOASTED HAZELNUTS AND BANANAS (SERVES 2)

*Breakfast is the most important meal of the day, and this great cereal will fuel your busy morning. Quick and easy to prepare, it can be eaten day in, day out, and if you use different fruits, nuts, and cereals every time you make it, you'll never get bored!*

2 cups bran flakes

2 Tbs. raisins or golden raisins

2 Tbs. mixed seeds (such as flax, hemp, sunflower, pumpkin, or sesame)

4 Tbs. toasted hazelnuts, roughly chopped

3 Tbs. banana chips, roughly chopped

Place the bran flakes in a bowl with the raisins, mixed seeds, hazelnuts, and banana chips. Thoroughly mix the ingredients together, then either eat immediately or store the cereal in an airtight container. When you're ready to enjoy it, add some chilled milk or yogurt, and, if you wish, sprinkle a selection of chopped fresh fruits over the top.

## *winning ways with granola*

- Stock up on granola ingredients such as oats, nuts, sunflower and pumpkin seeds, linseeds, dried fruits, shredded coconut, and plump golden raisins; store them in different jars. To help stave off granola boredom, throw different combinations together in the mornings.
- Toast nuts and seeds by spreading them on a baking tray and popping it under the broiler or in a hot oven for a few minutes (keeping an eagle eye on them to make sure that they turn golden brown rather than burning). They can then be kept in airtight storage jars.
- If you find granola a little tough, try soaking it in milk or apple juice overnight and topping it with sliced fresh fruits.

## CARDAMOM RICE MILK PORRIDGE (SERVES 2–3)

*One of the greatest advantages of owning a microwave is not having to wash a sticky pan after making porridge! You could also make this porridge with cow's, sheep's, goat's, or soy milk.*

3 oz. organic jumbo oats

1 1/4 cups rice milk

3 large green cardamom pods

clear honey, to taste

1 tsp. sesame seeds, toasted

In a bowl, mix the oats with the rice milk, then add the cardamom pods. Place in the microwave and zap on high for 90 seconds. Remove from the microwave and allow to settle for 1 minute. Next, remove and discard the cardamom pods and drizzle a little clear honey over the porridge. Sprinkle the sesame seeds on top and serve at once.

## CARROT AND ORANGE CAKE (MAKES AN 8-IN. CAKE)

*Getting a bit tired and in need of a lift? A piece of cake and a cup of tea always do the trick.*

1 cup butter

1 cup granulated brown sugar

4 eggs, beaten

zest and juice of 1 orange

1 1/3 cups whole-grain pastry flour

1 tsp. baking powder

7 oz. carrots, grated

1/2 cup ground almonds

*For the filling*

scant 1 1/4 cups light cream cheese

2 Tbs. confectioners' icing sugar

1/2 tsp. vanilla extract

Heat the oven to 350°. In a food processor, blend the butter and sugar until light and creamy. Gradually add the eggs, orange zest, and juice. Transfer to a bowl, then add the flour and baking powder. Stir in the carrots and almonds. Divide between two greased and lined 8-in. round cake pans. Bake for 30–40 minutes or until lightly golden. When cool enough to handle, turn out onto a wire rack. To serve, make a quick cream cheese filling by mixing together all the ingredients. Spread over one layer, and place other layer on top. Dust lightly with confectioners' sugar.

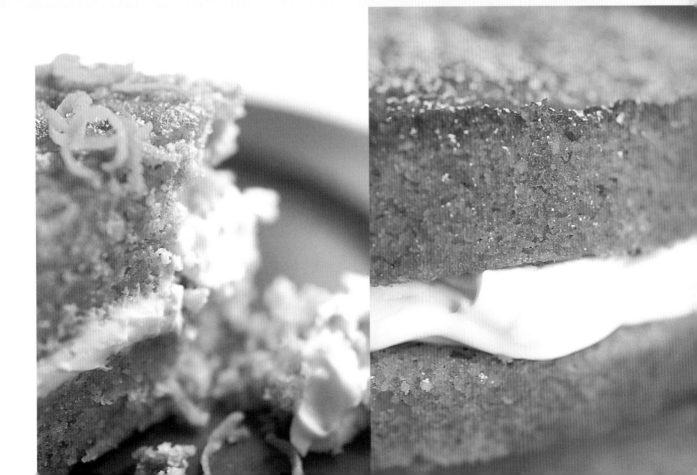

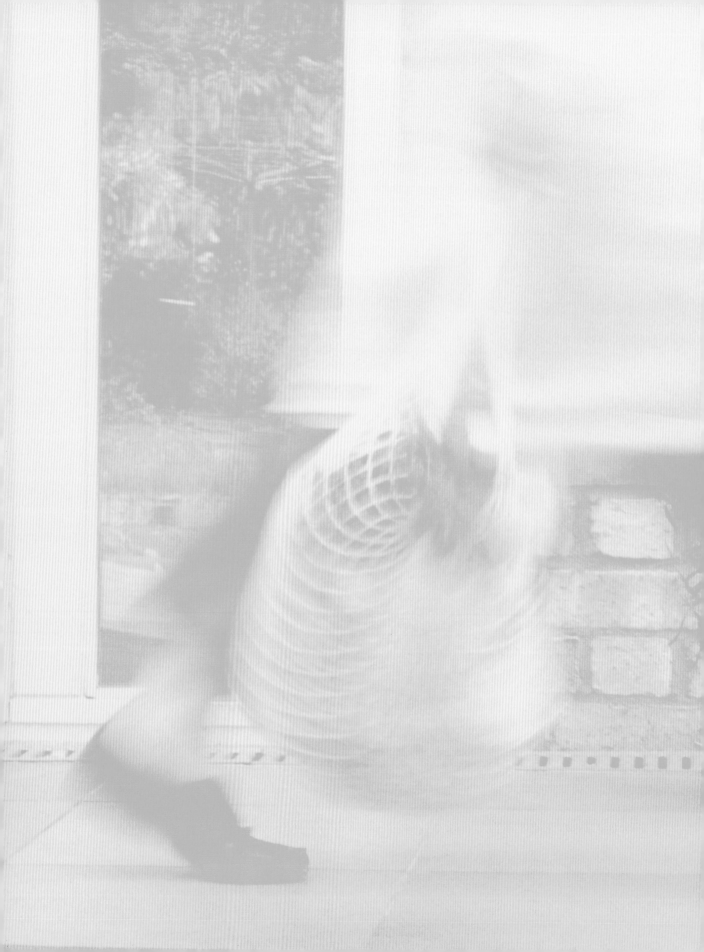

# bodyfoods
## practicalities

Understanding the principles of healthy eating is all well and good, but the problem for most of us is a lack of time, energy, and inclination to put those principles into practice. No, our busy lives certainly don't make eating well easy, and although there's some truth in my dad's frequent comment "Whoever said that anything was meant to be easy?" I've tried to show you in this chapter how you can make it less difficult for yourself.

# pantry staples

When time and energy are in short supply, it's important to put together a stash of essential ingredients that will stand you in good stead when you crave something to eat, but can't leave, or don't feel like leaving, the house.

Last week I gave my kitchen cupboards a thorough cleaning out, throwing out foodstuffs that hadn't been used for a year. It was a cathartic experience, but it also showed me just how much we store and then forget about, leaving lots of food to go to waste. If they're kept for too long, even teas and dried herbs can go off, especially in a nice warm kitchen. Although your pantry will, no doubt, reflect your personal tastes, the contents of mine may point you in the direction of some healthy options.

## essential ingredients for pantry meals

- Dried pasta, different shapes
- Rice, including risotto, long-grain, and wild rice
- Canned and dried legumes, including lentils, for chucking into soups and making dhal
- Canned baked beans for a last-minute, comforting supper
- Canned fish, such as dolphin-friendly tuna, salmon, sardines, and anchovies
- Oats for making oatmeal, granola, and oatmeal cookies
- Unsalted nuts, including hazelnuts and pine nuts, for roasting and adding to salads
- Seeds, including sunflower and pumpkin seeds
- Dried mushrooms for adding to risottos or making soup
- Dried fruits (organic, with no added $SO_2$), including raisins, apricots, and my favorite mangoes
- Dried herbs, such as bay, oregano, rosemary, and thyme, stored in dark, airtight containers
- Stock cubes
- Oils, including a good-quality olive oil for roasting vegetables and making salad dressings, a small bottle of fine, stronger-flavored olive oil for pouring neat over salads, and a nut oil, such as walnut or hazelnut, for enhancing dressings (use 1 part nut oil to 2 parts olive oil and 1 part vinegar)
- Vinegars, including white wine, balsamic, and special vinegars, such as my favorite walnut vinegar
- Soy sauce
- Jars of sun-blushed tomatoes, roasted artichokes, capers, anchovies, and olives
- Jars of mustards, tapenade, pesto, chutneys, and concentrated tomato sauce for jazzing up snacks
- Teas, both herbal and black teas (see pages 13 and 24–5)
- Crisp breads, including thin, Swedish crisp breads and savory, whole-wheat, oat-type crackers
- Eggs (ideally organic and stored at room temperature) for scrambling, poaching, and boiling

## 10 great standby suppers

1 Baked beans on toast or my favorite toasted baked bean and cheese sandwich: whole-wheat bread spread with a dollop of ketchup, laden with warmed baked beans and grated cheddar cheese, topped with another slice of bread, then toasted until golden and served with chutney.

2 An omelet made with a couple of eggs and filled with mushrooms, onions, olives, cheese, bacon, or any other leftovers from your fridge.

3 Slices of San Daniele or Parma ham, a few arugula leaves, lean salami, and a handful of capers make a terrific antipasto.

4 Canned salmon sandwich with cucumber, or mashed canned sardines with dill and a squeeze of lemon juice served on toast.

5 Quick and light mushroom soup, which is nourishing and easy to digest. Rinse $1/4$ cup dried porcino mushrooms and place in a bowl. Warm $2^{1}/_{2}$ pints chicken or vegetable stock and pour over the mushrooms. Leave for 10 minutes, then place in a saucepan to simmer for 30 minutes. Strain, then season and serve.

6 Pasta served with grated pecorino cheese, roasted pine nuts, a small piece of green chili (fried with a little garlic), plenty of black pepper, a touch of sea salt, and a good splash of extra-virgin olive oil.

7 Smoked mackerel pâté made by creaming some canned smoked mackerel fillets, cream cheese (1 Tbs. per mackerel fillet), and a squeeze of lemon juice. Serve with some hot whole-wheat toast and a bag of salad greens, if you have one.

8 Balls of fresh buffalo mozzarella, sliced and jazzed up with olive oil, balsamic vinegar, sea salt, and served with crisp breads.

9 Easy fried rice for two: heat a dash of peanut oil in your wok, add a couple of chopped green onions, and fry for a minute, then add a beaten egg. Throw in 2 cups cooked white rice, and fry for 2–3 minutes. Season with black pepper and a little sea salt.

10 Slices of pecorino cheese with pear and a prepackaged greens.

# fridge feasts

The phase "full fridge, full heart" definitely applies to me; I feel bereft when my fridge is empty. That said, we've all spent a small fortune stocking the fridge, only to have a change of plan that means the whole lot thrown into the garbage can—which may be why many working people keep their fridges sparsely filled.

The problem with keeping a virtually empty fridge is that when you are at home and hungry, but have no time to shop for food, you resort to a takeout or try to transform a can of tuna, which leaves you so unsatisfied that you end up tucking into that tub of ice cream, after all. The best strategy to stay healthy and in control of your working and home lives is to fill your fridge with staples that keep for a few days—or even weeks—and then occasionally bring home fresh ingredients, such as spinach leaves or salads, to jazz up your meals.

## tips for a happy, healthy fridge

- Keep your fridge between 32° and 41°. Regularly check the temperature with a thermometer
- Don't let raw meat or poultry come into contact with any cooked foods or those eaten raw, such as salads
- Keep all foods covered, but store cheese and eggs in non-airtight containers, so the air can circulate
- Defrost and clean your refrigerator regularly—festering fridges spell bad news for food!

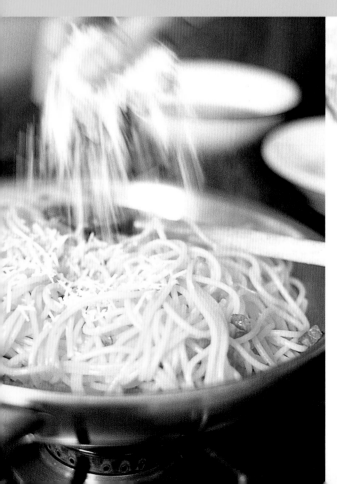
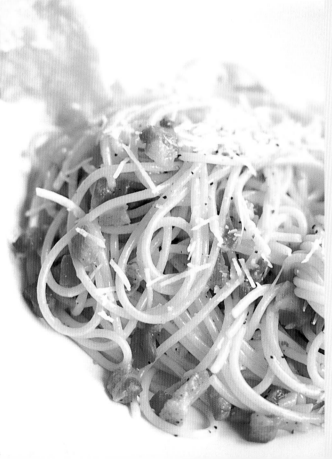

## favorite foods for a fully stocked fridge

- Butter
- Organic milk for serving chilled or warm with dates (see page 137), or for melting chocolate (with a minimum 70% cocoa solids) in—yummy!
- Cheese, both hard and soft, and always Parmesan. Take your cheese out of the fridge for an hour or so before eating; it will reward you with a much better flavor. Try my Pear, Pecorino, and Belgian endive Salad (see page 56) and Celery Sticks Stuffed with Goat Cheese and Chives (see page 74)
- Whole-milk yogurts, for adding to smoothies (see page 15), serving with fruit salads, such as my Fruit Confit in Spiced Syrup (see page 17), or adding to savory dishes, such as potato salad
- Strips of bacon for using in my Spaghetti with Eggs and Bacon (see page 62) and Chicken and Bacon Salad (see page 114). Add it to risottos, or eat it broiled with crispy baked potatoes
- Prosciutto and other cuts of cold, lean cooked meat
- Smoked salmon or mackerel, for using in sandwiches—it's delicious with dill, a squeeze of lemon, and a thin scraping of cream cheese (I'd use full fat, as the low fat is inferior tasting) inside fresh wholegrain bread
- Onions
- Garlic
- Olives
- Capers
- Squashes: I like just roasted squash drizzled with olive oil, a little sea salt, and plenty of black pepper as a comfort vegetable—or you could chop it up, roasted, in salads
- Tomatoes: take them out of the fridge a good hour before eating, as the cold flattens their flavor. Roast to serve with mozzarella (see page 56), or use in salads, in sandwiches, on toast, or in sauces. Little cherry tomatoes are also a good savory snack, naturally low in calories
- Tomato-based pasta sauces, either homemade (see page 80) or a store-bought variety, can be used with pasta and some fresh herbs, or used to make my Ragù alla Bolognese (see page 52)
- Salsa verde or rossa, bought or homemade (see page 92)
- Pesto, bought or homemade, for adding to pasta, broiled vegetables, and even salad dressings (use only ¼ tsp., as it can be overpowering). Try a thin scraping in toasted wholewheat sandwiches
- Soups, ideally homemade, otherwise some fresh, deli-counter soups
- Fresh gingerroot, for grating in boiling water, as a tea to settle stomachs and get rid of colds
- Apples and pears
- Lemons and limes
- Avocados are a must in a salad. Don't worry about their high fat content; it's a good vegetable fat, and if you use them in salads, you tend to need less olive oil dressing to make them moist
- Pure-fruit spreads
- Decaffeinated coffee beans and some caffeinated coffee beans for your early-morning kick-start or for an addicted guest!

# freezable bodyfoods

A freezer can be a busy person's lifeline, because it keeps most perishable foods fresh for months—that is, as long as the temperature is kept at 0° or lower. Although different foods freeze in different ways (depending on their flavor and water content), if you follow your freezer manual's instructions and any food labels, and also defrost and clean your freezer regularly, you'll stay one step ahead of the game.

## frozen assets

- Sliced loaves of whole-wheat bread; divide the slices between separate freezer bags so that you can use just a few at a time without the whole loaf going stale
- Part-baked bread, uncooked ciabattas and naan bread
- Organic milk: although freezing can make milk separate, making it look as if it's spoiled, it just needs a good shake. I buy more milk than I need and preserve it in my freezer so that it's always on hand. Soy milk doesn't tend to freeze well
- Butter
- Berries: great when blended with yogurt to make wonderful smoothies, which you can enjoy all year round. I find it's the most economical way to make berry smoothies, as fresh can be so expensive. Also good stewed (or you could substitute other fruits, such as plums, see my Stewed Plums and Orange Yogurt on page 53).
- Chicken portions, chops, bacon, and fish for using with pasta sauces, adding to salads, or broiling and simply drizzling with a little olive oil and maybe some fresh herbs
- Puff pastry (it's just not worth making your own): for making quick apple pies by filling with sliced cooking apples, a little brown sugar, and maybe some cinnamon or nutmeg. You could also make a plum pie with poached plums
- Vegetables (such as spinach), beans (such as fava beans) and corn: frozen vegetables usually contain just as many, if not more, vitamins and minerals than fresh ones because they're typically frozen so soon after harvesting that there's little time for their nutrients to degrade. They steam well as long as you cook from frozen—and can also be used in pasta sauces, even ready-made ones, which you want to make a little different. Some vegetables freeze better than others: I find peas, corn, and beans among the best, while spinach, cauliflower, and broccoli tend to become mushy, so they're best in sauces, and spicy Indian dishes. Experiment to see which suit your taste

## freezable dishes for emergency meals

I try to stock my freezer with a few dishes that I've cooked from scratch, such as soups and casseroles. Not only does it take the same amount of time and effort to cook double or triple portions, but if you divide them between airtight plastic containers, you'll be able to enjoy meals in minutes. This is where the microwave (see pages 54–5) comes into its own. Because it defrosts frozen dishes in minutes, rather than hours, you can select the meal you want now, instead of having to think a day ahead.

## RAGÙ ALLA BOLOGNESE (MAKES ABOUT 3 CUPS, OR SERVES 8–10 WITH PASTA)

*Serve this sauce with spaghetti or any other favorite pasta, or use it to make my Lasagna Verde al Forno.*

1/4 cup olive oil

1 small onion, minced

1 stalk celery, trimmed and chopped

1/2 medium carrot, chopped

2 or 3 slices prosciutto, minced

2 chicken livers, minced

1 lb. ground chuck

sea salt and freshly ground black pepper

1/4 cup dry white wine

5/8 cup milk

5/8 cup beef, veal, or chicken stock

13/4 cups Italian plum tomato sauce

Heat the oil in a large saucepan. Add the onion and cook for 3 minutes or until soft, but not brown. Add the celery and carrot and cook for another 3 minutes. Add the prosciutto and chicken livers, and cook, stirring constantly, for 1 minute or until just cooked, but still a little pink. Add the ground chuck, and season to taste. Cook for 5 minutes or until just done, but not browned, breaking it up as it cooks. Add the wine and cook, stirring constantly, for 3 minutes or until evaporated. Reduce the heat. In a separate pan, heat the milk, then add to the meat. Cook, stirring occasionally, for 10 minutes or until evaporated. Heat the stock and tomato paste, then add to the sauce. Simmer gently over a low heat, stirring occasionally, for 2 1/2 hours. Season to taste.

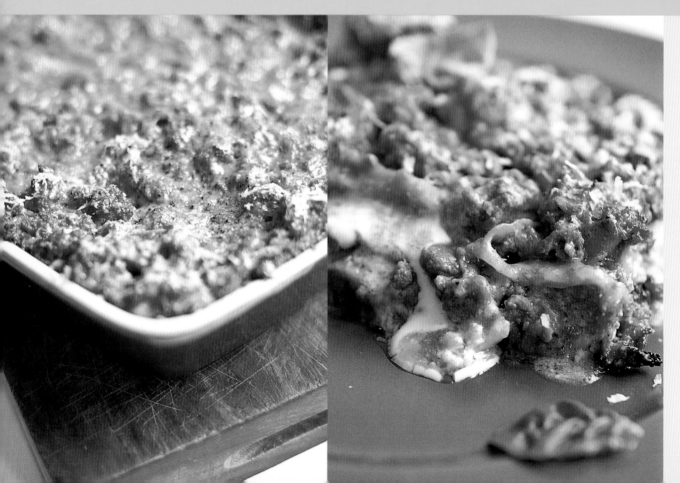

## LASAGNA VERDE AL FORNO (SERVES 8–12)

*Making lasagna can seem a hassle, but prepare it in advance and freeze it, or keep it in the fridge. Then, when you need a meal but have only an ounce of energy left, simply pop it in the oven to bake.*

2 Tbs. butter

5 sheets spinach pasta (6 x 22 in.)

3 cups Ragù alla Bolognese or ready-made
   bolognese sauce

9 oz. Parmesan cheese

2¹/₂ cups ready-made béchamel sauce

Heat the oven to 450°. Grease a 9- x 12-in. baking dish with the butter, and set aside. Bring a large pan of water to the boil, and add 2 generous pinches of salt. Cook the pasta, one sheet at a time, in the pan for 10 seconds or until it floats to the surface. Remove with a slotted spoon and plunge into salted, ice-cold water, to prevent further cooking. When each sheet has cooled, remove it from the water and lay it on damp paper towels. Cover with more damp paper towels. Do not let the pasta sheets touch each other. Line the bottom of the baking dish with a pasta sheet, trimming to fit (if necessary, patch any holes with pasta trimmings). Spread a third of the bolognese sauce evenly over the pasta, then lightly sprinkle some freshly grated Parmesan on top. Add another sheet of pasta, evenly spread half the béchamel sauce over it, then lightly sprinkle with more Parmesan. Continue until you have built up three layers of bolognese sauce and two of béchamel sauce, ending with a layer of bolognese sauce and Parmesan. Bake in the oven for 10 minutes, then increase the temperature to 475° and bake for another 5–7 minutes or until browned on top. Remove from the oven and allow to rest for 8–10 minutes before serving.

## STEWED PLUMS WITH ORANGE YOGURT (SERVES 2)

*In this recipe, which serves two, I have married the plums with some creamy sheep yogurt, making a delicious combination. If you can't get sheep yogurt, substitute low-fat Greek yogurt.*

¹/₂ lb. fresh plums

1 cup sheep yogurt, or low-fat Greek yogurt

juice of 1 orange

finely grated rind of half the orange

¹/₂ Tbs. fine granulated sugar

Stone the plums. Place them in a large saucepan and sprinkle with the sugar. Cover the pan, place it over a low heat, and leave the plums to stew for 3 to 4 minutes. Leaving the pan covered, turn off the heat and let the plums stand for 10 to 12 minutes to continue to soften. Transfer the plums to a sieve set over a bowl to allow their juices to drain away. Now tip the plums into a bowl and leave them to cool completely. Meanwhile, mix the orange juice and rind with the yogurt. Lightly crush the plums with a fork to make them more of a purée, then gently swirl them into the yogurt to create an attractive marbled effect. Spoon the dessert into two glasses, and serve with some ginger cookies.

# microwave meals

Over the past decade, the microwave has been promoted from a gadget that was occasionally used to heat up a cooked dish to many people's main cooking appliance. Because microwaving takes only minutes, dirties no pans, and can transform a package pulled from the freezer into a hearty meal in the time it takes to have a quick shower, some people never feel the need to turn on the oven.

Although I appreciate being able to produce a meal in minutes, I wish fewer people relied so heavily on microwaves, because they're depriving themselves of the pleasurable aspects of cooking: the smells, flavors, colors and textures that only oven cooking bestows. Our busy lives make microwaves a necessity; but, having accepted that, I'd still urge you to use yours sparingly—perhaps for scrambling eggs, heating up your bedtime milk, or the occasional ready-prepared meal, for example. Use your microwave, but use it well.

## are there are any benefits to using a microwave?

The microwave does offer some distinct nutritional advantages, particularly when it comes to vegetables, which the microwave cooks in a short time without the need for much water. This means nutrients don't leach out into the water, as they do when vegetables are boiled. Microwaved or steamed green, leafy vegetables, like spinach, contain more vitamin C than their boiled counterparts. If the smell of cooking fish puts you off, using the microwave is a good option, because it will contain much of the odor. And if the speed of microwave cooking means that you'll eat something healthful, instead of having a greasy takeout or a huge bag of potato chips and some chocolate last thing at night, then it's a good thing.

## are microwaves dangerous?

There has been much speculation in the press that microwaves are bad for our health, with scary words like "irradiation" and "carcinogenic" being bandied about. Don't be put off: microwaving is a safe way of cooking, as long as you follow the manufacturer's instructions regarding both the microwave and the cooking of microwavable dishes. There are, however, two pitfalls that are vital to avoid:

1 Cold spots are small areas that are missed by the microwaves, within which bacteria may then breed, causing food poisoning. Reduce this likelihood by making sure that the turntable rotates freely and isn't overloaded. When cooking a number of items at once, make sure they are of a similar size, so that it is easier to calculate when the microwave has heated all of the food to the point needed to kill the bad bacteria.

2 It's important to leave large pieces of food, such as joints of meat, to stand after the microwave cooking time, to allow the residual heat to penetrate the center, ensuring that the food is evenly cooked throughout. If standing time is required, it should be clearly stated in your microwave manual or on the food label.

## tips for making the most of your microwave

- Microwaves currently vary in wattage from 400 to 1,000 watts. The lower the wattage, the longer food will take to cook, so it may be worth investing in a high-wattage appliance

- Don't try to hard-boil eggs or cook shellfish (because they might explode), turkey, or smoked ham (their salt content will make them shrivel up) or batter-based dishes (the results look really unappetizing)

- Always cover food to ensure faster, more even cooking (successful microwaving involves a combination of the action of the microwaves and the heat of the steam, which also tenderizes food). You don't, however, need to cover dry, crisp foods like cookies. If you're microwaving bread, wrap it in a paper towel, which will soak up excess moisture and stop the bread from becoming soggy, and remove the paper as soon as you take the bread out of the microwave

- If food is unevenly shaped, arrange it so that the thicker part is in the center (microwaved food cooks from the inside out)

- Arrange equal-sized pieces evenly on the plate, and leave gaps between them

- If the food is covered with a tight skin or membrane, like many vegetables, pierce the skin with a fork

- Make sure that you stir or turn the food at regular intervals, while it is cooking, to encourage the heat to permeate every part

- If food is cooking too fast, check that your power level isn't set too high. Another cause may be that the oven has a higher wattage than the recipe requires, in which case adjust the cooking time

- If food is cooking too slowly, check that your power level is set correctly. Alternatively, the food may have been at the wrong temperature when you put it in the microwave (fish, poultry, meat, and most vegetables should be at refrigerator temperature, while dry goods and canned foods should be at room temperature). Or does your microwave share a circuit with another appliance? If so, it may not be operating at full power. Finally, you may not have left the food to stand for the recommended time, as this is part of the cooking process

# everyday packed lunches

Here are some dishes that both travel well and taste great—no soggy sandwiches or limp salads, I promise! Remember, it's best to keep all home-prepared food refrigerated for as long as possible before leaving home to minimize the risk of contamination by food-poisoning bacteria.

## PEAR, PECORINO, AND BELGIAN ENDIVE SALAD (SERVES 1)

*Belgian endive stays crunchy in lunchbox salads. It combines beautifully with pear and pecorino.*

Wash and core 1 ripe pear, then slice into 8 pieces. Slice the base off 1 endive head, then separate the leaves. Arrange the endive leaves and pear slices in an airtight plastic container. Drizzle over a little olive oil and balsamic vinegar. Season with lots of black pepper and top with some shavings of pecorino cheese.

## LEEK AND BACON FLAN (SERVES 6–8)

*Quiches and flans keep well in airtight plastic containers, providing a tasty, lighter option to the sandwich.*

9-in. unbaked pastry shell (preferably whole-grain) in quiche pan

4 Tbs. butter

4 strips lean bacon, chopped into small pieces

1 lb. leeks, washed and sliced into rings

3 organic free-range eggs, beaten

$5/8$ cup whole milk

1 tsp. Dijon mustard

$4^{1}/2$ oz. Gruyère cheese, grated

sea salt and freshly ground black pepper

Heat the oven to 375°. Line a 9-in. quiche pan with the pastry. Line the pastry with waxed paper, weight it down with baking beans, and bake the flan case in the oven for 8–10 minutes, or until the pastry starts to turn a pale-golden color. Melt the butter in a skillet, add the bacon, and fry until golden. Now add the leeks, and fry until they become soft, transparent, and slightly golden in color. Remove the pan from the heat, and transfer the bacon mixture to the flan case, spreading it evenly over the bottom. Beat the eggs, then stir in the milk, mustard, and cheese. Season with a little sea salt and plenty of freshly ground black pepper. Pour the egg filling into the flan case, place it in the oven, and bake for about 30 minutes, or until the top is golden brown. Once the flan has cooled, cut it into slices.

## ROASTED TOMATO AND MOZZARELLA SALAD (SERVES 1)

*I like to team this salad with some Swedish rye crackers or a lightly buttered wholewheat roll.*

Heat the oven to 375°. Place a couple of large handfuls of ripe cherry tomatoes in a roasting pan with a sprig of rosemary and a large dash of olive oil. Sprinkle with a little sea salt and freshly ground black pepper. Roast in the oven for about 30 minutes or until softened and starting to brown. Remove from the oven to cool. Tear a buffalo mozzarella into medium-sized pieces and place in a small airtight plastic container, along with the cooled tomatoes. Drizzle with a little fresh olive oil, and sprinkle with some torn, fresh basil.

## CAESAR SALAD-FILLED ROLLS (SERVES 1)

*This is a great way of making a portable sandwich with a delicious dressing.*

*For the dressing*

1 Tbs. mayonnaise

1 small garlic clove, crushed

2 Tbs. finely grated Parmesan cheese

sea salt and freshly ground black pepper

1 large wholewheat roll

2 anchovy fillets

1 small egg, hard-boiled and chopped

1 Tbs. roughly chopped parsley

romaine leaves, trimmed and chopped

Mix the mayonnaise with enough water to make a pourable dressing. Add the garlic, Parmesan, and plenty of seasoning. Halve one large wholewheat roll, and scoop out a little of the crumb from each half. Drizzle with a little of the dressing, then top the bottom half with the anchovy fillets, egg, parsley, and lettuce. Drizzle the remainder of the dressing over, and top with the other half roll. Wrap in waxed paper or foil.

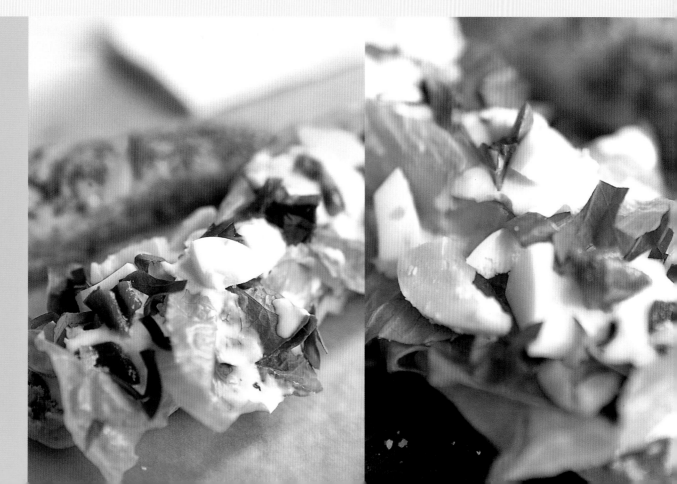

# energy-boosting snacks

We spend so many hours working to keep on top of our busy lives that our bodies can find it difficult to maintain the energy levels and concentration required on just three meals a day. Not only do we feel, and perform, better if we refuel with a few judiciously chosen snacks; they also ward off the extreme hunger pangs that frequently drive us to eat too much, too quickly, and often unhealthily. Having a little nutritious something mid-morning or late afternoon can, by contrast, make meal times body-nurturing affairs.

The secret lies in picking the right snacks. Give a wide berth to those that aggravate digestive problems, encourage you to pile on the pounds, or send your blood-sugar level, and consequently moods, shooting up and down. High-fat, high-sugar snacks like candy bars, potato chips, cookies and carbonated drinks are the worst offenders, and, unfortunately, the most easily obtainable. When deciding which snack will help, not hinder, your body, look for two or three key ingredients: fruit and fiber, followed by protein.

The best snacks to buy are fresh or dried fruits (with no added sulfur dioxide or syrupy coating, and have only a few), unsalted nuts, roasted-seed mixes, and small tubs of yogurt. Other options include chunks of cheese with celery, whole or oat-based wheat- or crisp breads to team with a little cheese (maybe soft goat cheese), or slices of cold meat (like prosciutto) and a few cherry tomatoes—perhaps you could keep a supply of ingredients in the fridge at work. Whatever you eat, remember to sip plenty of water while nibbling.

## snack satisfaction

Sometimes we think that we want food when, in fact, it's a drink we need (your brain may simply require oral satisfaction, but its message may have become confused). If your desire to snack is spiraling out of control, have a glass of water, a cup of good-quality tea, or an herbal infusion, and you may just find that it does the trick. Taking the time to present your snack attractively and then savoring it also send messages of satiety to your brain, unlike constantly grazing, which bamboozles it into thinking that your stomach's never satisfied.

Indeed, it's much preferable to concentrate on enjoying your snacks—regard them as opportunities to take a break and clear your head—rather than grabbing something to eat while you're on the go, which can cause indigestion, bloating, and, ultimately, weight gain. If it is to produce the right digestive enzymes, your body also needs to be given the chance to register that you've eaten, and if you're dashing around, it's too busy focusing on your muscles to digest your snack properly. If you've got the time to cook ahead, or have access to a kitchen at work, here are a few ideas for some more energizing snacks.

## SPICED ROASTED NUTS AND SEEDS

*Nuts and seeds contain omega oils and protein, which provide a long-lasting energy boost. Make up a large batch (about 4 cups) of your favorite nuts and seeds, and then carry a pack around with you to nibble at work, or at home in front of the television. They keep in an airtight jar for up to three weeks.*

Heat the oven to 400°. Use your favorite nuts and seeds, following my recipe as a guide. Place 1 cup each of blanched almonds, cashew nuts, unsalted peanuts, and walnuts in a bowl. Sprinkle 2 Tbs. sesame seeds, 3 Tbs. pumpkin seeds and 3 Tbs. sunflower seeds on top. Add 2 Tbs. olive oil, 1 Tbs. clear honey, 1 tsp. chili flakes, and a large pinch each of ground coriander and ground cumin. Mix all the ingredients until coated in the oil. Spread evenly over a baking tray, and roast in the oven for 5–10 minutes or until light golden, turning them halfway through. Remove from the oven, add some sea salt, and leave to cool completely; then seal in a clean jar.

## A TAPAS PLATTER

*This is the ideal way to entertain friends if you have only the time and energy to do a one-hit shop and would prefer to spend the few precious moments before they arrive getting yourself ready.*

Select your ingredients either from your supermarket's delicatessen counter or, better still, a Spanish deli. Allow 3 or 4 slices of cold meat (such as chorizo and Serrano ham) per person, and arrange on a large platter. Place slices of Manchego cheese alongside the cold meats. Manchego is traditionally served with quince jelly (*membrillo*), the perfect accompaniment. Fill dishes with pickled chilies, olives, sweet pickles, sun-kissed tomatoes, roasted peppers, mushrooms, or artichokes. Serve your tapas platter with a large bowl of ready-prepared herb salad and some warmed, fresh, crusty bread.

## CHERRY AND COCONUT ENERGIZING BARS (MAKES 12)

*These bars are a great energy-boosting standby. Remove them from the oven while still slightly soft, as they will harden up on cooling and make a delicious moist, chewy bar.*

1 1/2 sticks butter

5 Tbs. corn syrup

1/4 cup granulated brown sugar

1 1/4 cups rolled oats

1 1/8 cups barley flakes

5/8 cups shredded coconut

scant 1/2 cup dried sour cherries

Heat the oven to 350°. In a large pan, melt the butter with the corn syrup and sugar. Stir well, then add all the remaining ingredients. Spoon into a greased 9- x 12-in. cake pan, and bake in the oven for 20 minutes or until lightly golden. Leave to cool slightly, then score into 12 bars. Leave to cool completely in the pan before eating.

# bodyfoods solutions
# for eating late

Eating late is part and parcel of our busy lives. Very few of us have the time in which to prepare, and eat, a meal at 5:30 P.M.–I certainly don't get back from work and finish writing until at least 8 P.M., and some evenings it's way past 9 P.M., at which point it's crucial to choose the foods that will help me sleep.

The worst thing you can do when it's late is not eat anything at all, because the result of depriving your body of nourishment until the morning will most likely be waking up feeling completely exhausted before you've even gotten going. You should always try to eat something in the evening to enable your body to replenish the reserves of vitamins, minerals, and other essential nutrients that it's been drawing on during the day. If you don't, your blood-sugar level will plummet during the night, and you'll wake up feeling drained, weak, and ratty.

## late-night comfort foods

Foods that sit best in the stomach when you're eating late are those that aren't too hard to digest. Avoid fatty, rich, creamy, and fried foods or lots of raw vegetables or fruits, which are simply too much of a challenge for your digestive system to cope with at this time. You're much better off having a simple carbohydrate-, starch-based meal or snack—such as a bowl of pasta with a simple sauce, a baked potato, or some rice teamed with a stir-fry—which will not only be relatively easy to digest (as long as it's not saturated with too much oil or too many spices), but also make you feel well fed and nurtured, not stuffed. Because such meals encourage the brain to produce endorphins ("happy" hormones), they trigger a childlike response to having a full, warm stomach, namely a contented, soporific feeling which is ideal at the end of a stressful day.

My favorite late-night supper is baked beans, which, if I'm well organized, I've made myself (see page 33), although the canned alternatives are good substitutes. For me, little can beat beans on wholewheat toast as a comforting meal, especially when topped with a little cheddar. Beans are high in vegetable protein, the tomato sauce provides some lycopene, while both the beans and wholewheat toast contain fiber. Eggs or cheese on toast are other meals that have been ditched simply for reasons of fashion. Yet, they're nutritious, economical, and easy to make and, most importantly, sit comfortably in a tired and stressed stomach.

You may find that having a solitary chunk of cheese straight from the fridge disturbs your stomach and consequently your dreams, which is why it's better to incorporate it into a meal. Some people also find that having a meal that's based on protein and vegetables alone, such as a steak and salad, can have such a stimulating effect that it's impossible to wind down quickly enough to drop off to sleep. Red meat also tends to be very hard to digest, so you're better off having white meat, like chicken, or a little fish.

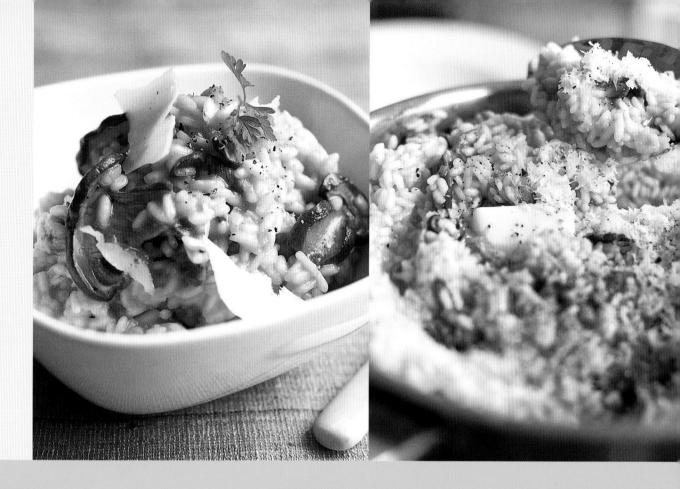

## 5 ways to avoid feeling lousy in the morning

1 Have a late-afternoon snack (such as fresh fruit, dried fruits, a whole-wheat cookie, a yogurt or a smoothie) to ensure that you won't be so ravenous on getting home that you eat anything and everything in sight.

2 Your favorite tipple can unwind you, but do not drink on an empty stomach. Eat something to keep the alcohol in your stomach for longer and ward off blood-sugar and energy crashes that leave you too tired to eat well.

3 Drink a couple of large glasses of water on getting home, to rehydrate your body. This will both minimize the negative effects of alcohol and help you to gauge how hungry you really are. Avoid drinking caffeine too late in the day, and have a relaxing, digestion-soothing herbal tea (see page 13) instead.

4 Avoid very sugary foods late at night, because they'll give you a sugar and energy high just when you want to drift into a deep slumber. The best types of sugar to eat at night are those provided by fresh fruits, which the body absorbs slowly. Similarly, avoid overly spicy or fatty dishes.

5 Pasta, rice, potatoes, and other starchy foods encourage the body to produce sleep-inducing hormones. Opt for a sauce that isn't too heavy. Instead of a creamy one, have a tomato sauce accompanied by a little (not a lot of) pecorino, mozzarella, or Parmesan cheese, and some lean bacon or prosciutto, rather than fatty salami.

# speedy late-night suppers

## SPAGHETTI WITH EGGS AND BACON (SERVES 4)

*Falling through the door late requires nourishment in minutes, using ingredients that are in your fridge and cabinets. This favorite comfort dish is for times when work seems to dominate your life.*

9 oz. pancetta or unsmoked bacon

1 garlic clove, lightly crushed

3 eggs, beaten

sea salt and freshly ground black pepper

3 Tbs. Parmesan cheese

3 Tbs. pecorino cheese

14 oz. spaghetti

In a large pan, fry the pancetta or bacon in its own fat. Add the garlic and cook until well browned. Remove and discard the garlic. Either remove the pan from the heat or turn the heat right down. To the beaten eggs add a pinch of sea salt, plenty of freshly ground black pepper, and 1 Tbs. each of the Parmesan and pecorino cheeses. In the meantime, cook the spaghetti in plenty of boiling, salted water for roughly 10 minutes or until the pasta is al dente. Drain the spaghetti thoroughly, transfer it to the bacon pan, stir well, and then remove from the heat. Stir in the egg mixture to form a fluid, yellow cream, then add the remaining Parmesan and pecorino and stir again. Transfer to hot plates and serve immediately.

## CRISP, CHEESE-FILLED BAKED POTATO (SERVES 1)

*With a little imagination the humble baked potato can become a suppertime star. The way I do them allows you to stir any ingredients into the soft, fluffy potato flesh, which I then spoon back into the skin, finishing off with a broiling to crisp the filling up. This recipe makes a satisfying meal for one. When you can't wait for an hour, cook the baked potato in the microwave first until soft, stuff, and then place under the hot broiler to crisp it. Be warned, though; the taste won't be quite as good.*

Heat the oven to 400°. Wash, scrub, and prick one baking potato. Place it in the oven for approximately 1 hour, or until it is tender in the middle and crisp on the outside. Remove the potato from the oven and cut it in half. Scoop out all of the soft potato flesh, and transfer it to a bowl. Stir in 2 Tbs. soft cream cheese, 2 finely chopped green onions, and, if you have any fresh herbs on hand, maybe 1 Tbs. chopped chives or parsley. Season to taste with freshly ground black pepper and sea salt. Then spoon the mixture back into the potato skins, place them on a baking tray and sprinkle 2 Tbs. grated or crumbled cheese of your choice (one of my favorites is Roquefort) on top. Place the baking tray under a hot broiler, and leave the cheese-and-potato mixture to melt and crisp up for a couple of minutes. Enjoy immediately with a freshly prepared salad or, for a more substantial supper, perhaps some sausages and baked beans.

*favorite combinations for late meals in 10 minutes*

Although early in the evening is the healthiest time to have a meal at the end of the day, this is often impossible for busy people. When you're eating late, it's important to choose those foods that will nurture, not overload, your body, enabling you to get a good night's sleep. Here are some of my favorites.

- Torn slivers of lean ham, such as prosciutto, peas (frozen are fine), very finely chopped shallots and garlic (sauté both lightly), fresh mint, and a pinch of freshly crushed coriander seeds
- Mozzarella, with small, ripe, cherry tomatoes, basil, and a little finely chopped fresh chili pepper
- Ready roasted chicken, with sage, olives, artichoke hearts, and olive oil
- Smoked salmon, with capers, dill, and a dollop of sour cream
- Sun-dried tomatoes (torn into small pieces), with basil, fresh tomatoes, and goat cheese
- A bowl of delicatessen fresh soup (avoid creamy ones, which can be difficult to digest late at night), with whole-wheat bread or toast, and perhaps a little cheese (mozzarella goes well with tomato soup)
- Yogurt with fruit, or a bowl of bananas with custard—although these don't offer all the essentials a proper meal should contain, milk-based foods, such as yogurt and custard, do contain trytophan, which encourages the brain to produce sleep-nurturing endorphins
- Pasta, with cottage cheese, a teaspoon of chopped fresh herbs, a smidge of tarragon mustard, seasoned with a little sea salt and black pepper—real comfort food

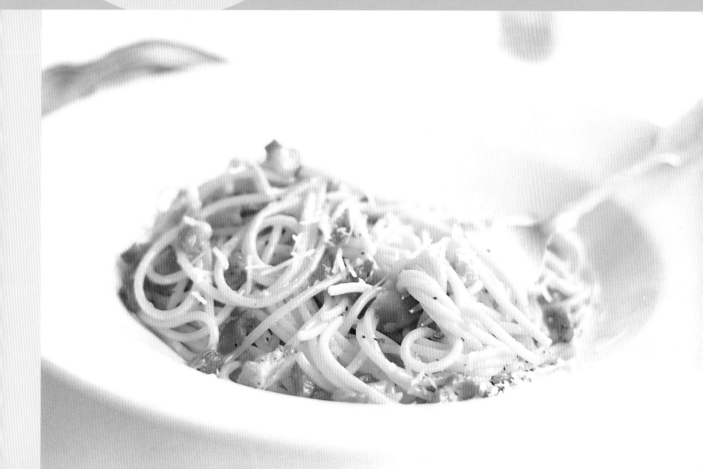

## ITALIAN BEANS WITH PASTA (SERVES 4)

*Ready in minutes, this is a hearty pantry recipe. If you can't find borlotti beans, use cannellini (also called white kidney beans). Penne is a good pasta to use, as the sauce coats its shape beautifully.*

1 Tbs. olive oil

1 red onion, chopped

2 garlic cloves, crushed

4 oz. pancetta or bacon, chopped

1 Tbs. fresh thyme or rosemary, chopped

2$^1$/$_2$ cups canned borlotti or cannellini beans

1 cup vegetable or chicken stock

14 oz. dried pasta, such as penne

Heat the olive oil in a pan, add the onion, garlic, and pancetta and fry for 3–4 minutes. Stir in the thyme or rosemary. Drain and rinse the beans, then stir them into the onion mixture. Pour the stock over and bring to the boil. Cover the pan and leave to simmer for 10 minutes. Meanwhile, bring a large pan of salted water to the boil, drop in the pasta and cook according to the instructions on the package. Using a slotted spoon, remove a quarter of the bean mixture from the pan, transfer it to a bowl, and set aside. Pour the remaining bean mixture into a blender and blend until it is smooth. Season to taste with freshly ground black pepper and sea salt, then pour the bean sauce back into the pan, also adding the reserved beans and 2 Tbs. chopped fresh parsley. Season to taste with more freshly ground black pepper and sea salt. Drain the pasta, stir in the sauce, and serve.

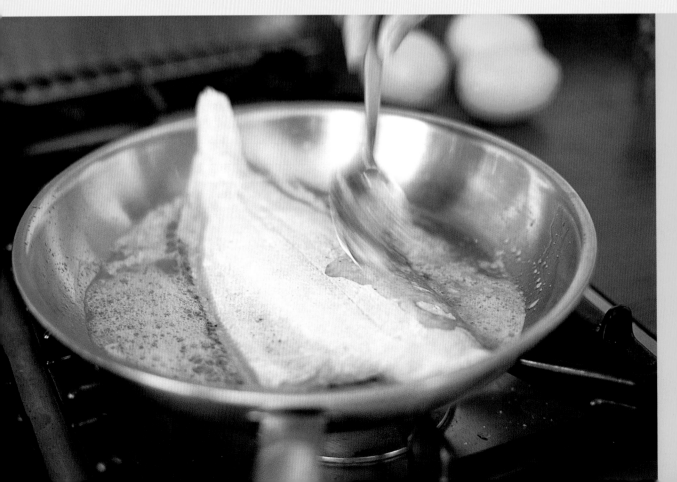

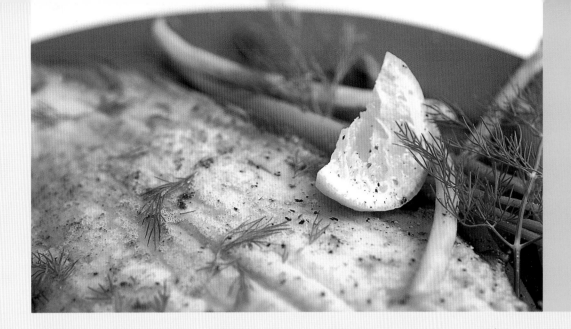

## PAN-FRIED SOLE (SERVES 1)

*If the idea of cooking fish is daunting, rest assured that it's as easy as pie. Although frying is traditionally unhealthful, this is a fish that's best cooked quickly to avoid drying out, and if you serve it with fresh vegetables, it's a quick, easy, and healthful supper. If you can't get sole, use flounder. Dusting it in flour before frying it gives a light, crisp crust; alternatively, fry it in a little butter over a high heat, sprinkle some chopped fresh herbs on top, and squeeze some lemon juice over.*

Melt 4 Tbs. butter in a large skillet over medium heat. Meanwhile, dip 1 large sole fillet in a little milk to wet its surface, then dip it into some flour seasoned with sea salt and freshly ground black pepper. When the butter starts to foam, carefully lay the fish in the butter and then leave it alone for 2–3 minutes. Using a large spatula, carefully turn over the fillet and fry the other side until it is crisp and golden. Lift the fillet out of the pan and transfer it to a warmed serving plate. Add a small knob of butter to the pan and, as soon as it has melted, pour it over the fish. Squeeze some lemon juice over the fish and enjoy at once with some freshly steamed vegetables.

## INDIAN SPICED SCRAMBLED EGGS (SERVES 2)

*A favorite of the family I frequently stay with when I visit India—a comforting, substantial meal.*

Melt 1/2 Tbs. butter in a skillet. Add 1 finely chopped small onion, 1/2-in. piece ginger, peeled and grated, and 1 fresh hot chili (optional), deseeded and minced. Cook for about 5 minutes, until the onion turns golden. Add 1/2 tsp. ground cumin and 1/2 tsp. ground turmeric, and fry for 1 minute then add 2 chopped tomatoes. After a couple more minutes of stirring over the heat, add 4 beaten organic eggs. Season to taste with a little sea salt and freshly ground black pepper, and throw in 2 Tbs. chopped fresh cilantro leaves. Serve, while the eggs are still runny.

# bodyfoods solutions for takeouts and fast foods

Occasionally we all find ourselves with no alternative but to eat fast food. There are many different types, however, and if you make an informed choice, fast food needn't affect you too badly. That said, fast foods are seldom the best option for your body and should be regarded as emergency fuel. If you manage to eat well most of the time, a fast-food fix needn't hit you hard. One damage-limitation strategy is to order a bottle of water to drink, to help your body deal with the undesirable nutrients, such as salt, that these foods contain.

## pizzas

As long as you don't have a problem digesting wheat, pizza can be a good choice. Those topped with lean ham, chicken, or plain tomatoes are more healthful than those containing salami and a number of cheeses, which are usually high in fat. Variety is the spice of life, so ask for your pizza to be divided into sections, perhaps with a third topped with ham, a third with mushrooms and peppers, and plain tomatoes on the remaining third? This will be far more satisfying than a single-flavor pizza. Order a side salad, but either have it plain or opt for a yogurt or vinaigrette dressing rather than a creamy, mayonnaise-based one. Lay off the garlic bread; and, because thick crusts tend to be difficult to digest, a thin-crust pizza is a preferable option.

## burgers

In theory, a burger made with broiled or grilled, lean meat wedged into a simple bun should be reasonably healthful. In practice the meat is usually high in fat (the burgers having been fried rather than broiled or grilled) and it tends to be teamed with a portion of very thin French fries, which have a higher fat-to-potato ratio than thick ones. As if this almighty dose of fat and calories isn't enough, the final insult is typically a mayonnaise-based dressing and the accompaniment of a cola drink or a thick milk shake, loaded with sugar. It's best to skip the French fries altogether and to choose a fish, chicken, or veggie "burger," all of which are a little lower in fat than meat burgers. None can be considered a healthful choice, however, just a better one.

## Tex-Mex

As tasty as their menu is, watch that you don't end up piling an awful lot of saturated fat into your stomach along with the Jalapeno peppers—even lighter choices, such as a chicken sandwich, can contain two cheeses, taking the saturated fat intake and calorie total right up. This can be made even heavier on your gut if you then tuck into the refried beans, sour cream, and guacamole. Less is more with Tex-Mex; ask for dressings and sauces to be served on the side, so you can control how much goes onto your meat and in your tortillas. Don't think that just because a free refill is offered with the soft drinks and iced tea that you can get away with drinking lots with no consequences—both soft drinks and iced tea contain loads of sugar, which can lead to tooth decay, energy level problems, weight gain and even headaches. Drink plenty of water instead.

## hotdogs

Nothing like as delicious as a homemade hot dog, made with a good-quality sausage and fresh bread, the fast-food hot dog leaves much to be desired. Almost all varieties contain sodium nitrite, which some researchers allege are carcinogens, although others deny this. Sodium nitrite is a chemical salt used as a preservative and flavor enhancer. It is particularly effective against botulism strains. People watching their fat intake can choose low-fat (one to nine grams of fat and 50 to 110 calories) and fat-free (less than a half gram of fat and 35 to 40 calories) weiners or switch to vegetarian tofu franks. Beware choosing chicken or turkey hot dogs in order to reduce your fat intake, as these are not always lower in fat. Unfortunately, fat-free dogs won't have the flavor of regular ones; cutting out fat means cutting a lot of the flavor and texture. As to the sauces and pickles— mustards and ketchups are frequently loaded with sugar and preservatives, and the pickles send the salt barometer sky high; so keep these to a minimum. The same applies to the high-calorie fried onions.

## submarine sandwiches

Some are so enormous, they're really big enough for two—so why not share one with a friend? Filling-wise, keep the mayo and relishes down to a minimum, as these can be very high in sugar and preservatives.

## Indian food

If, like me, you're frequently tempted, spare yourself indigestion and excess calories by opting for dishes with a tomato or stock base, chicken and seafood curries, and plain rice. Meat dishes, creamy kormas, and those made with coconut milk and fried rice are the heaviest. Naans contain less fat than chapattis, but poppadoms, samosas, and bhajis are dripping in it. Choosing several dishes, or side orders of pickles, gives you different taste sensations. Bean and lentil dishes are good stomach-fillers, so include both of these in your meal.

## Chinese food

Avoid a fat and monosodium glutamate (MSG) overload by choosing dim sum, steamed ribs, fish and chicken, stir-fries, plain rice, and vegetables (such as water chestnuts, Chinese broccoli, and greens). Duck, glutinous sauces, like sweet and sour, and fried dough balls hit the stomach hard (steamed ones are better for you).

## Japanese and Thai food

The Japanese cuisine is one of the lightest and most healthful, focusing as it does on fresh ingredients, including raw fish, rice noodles, soups, vegetables, and stir-fries (which are cooked to order over a high heat). Because it consists of lots of soups, chili, lemongrass, non-dairy foods, and noodle-based dishes, Thai food can also be a healthy option. The Thai style of eating, involving a variety of small, tasty dishes, can result in maximum satiety—just don't be tempted to order too many! If you suffer from heartburn, avoid green curries and chili-loaded dishes. Coconut curries tend to be somewhat rich, and meat dishes rather fatty, so order chicken, seafood, or vegetable-based dishes instead, and steamed rice rather than fried. As with all Chinese and Indian restaurants that serve rice, you should scrutinize your fast-food outlet for cleanliness, because both raw fish and rice can harbor food-poisoning bacteria.

# bodyfoods solutions for eating in restaurants

Eating out used to be something that was done mainly on special occasions, but restaurants (along with fast-food outlets, see pages 66–7) seem to have become the equivalent of many people's personal dining rooms, at least on a few occasions a week. This means that the old tradition that eating in a restaurant gives us *carte blanche* to indulge ourselves with a lavish meal is no longer appropriate, for if we did it regularly, we'd quickly become overweight.

Although I love eating out, and do so regularly, I try to balance succumbing to temptation with choosing the foods that will suit my body. Indeed, eating out can be extremely healthy, especially now that many restaurant menus offer plenty of lighter eating options. Here are some nutritional tricks of the trade to help you to order the right foods for your body at any time of day.

## breakfast

Many people feel more alert after eating a protein- and fruit-based breakfast—for example, grilled bacon with mushrooms and eggs, prosciutto with melon or figs, smoked salmon, or a fresh-fruit salad with yoghurt— rather than pastries, pancakes, sugary cereals, or mounds of toast (if you have toast, request wholewheat). Although a cup of good-quality coffee or tea can wake you up, it can make you feel anxious and stressed too, so if you're feeling jittery, consider ordering herbal tea (see page 13). Having a large breakfast may make you feel sluggish, so it's best not to overindulge, and if you have enjoyed a large breakfast, eat a lighter lunch.

## lunch

Some people feel sleepy after eating a starchy meal, which is usually the last thing you need in the middle of the day. So if you're lunching out, limit your intake of pasta, rice, potatoes, couscous, and bread. Light dishes like chicken, fish, omelets, sushi, sashimi, stir-fries, or cold cuts with simple salads or broiled vegetables are generally better suited to lunchtime eating than the richer, French-style, sauce-based cuisine. Before ordering, take into consideration what you'll be eating in the evening to avoid hitting your body with two large meals. Steer clear of alcohol, which can hit your body doubly hard at this time of day.

## dinner

If you have a table for late in the evening, try to have a substantial snack (see pages 58–9) toward the end of the afternoon to avoid feeling so ravenous by the time you get to the restaurant that you end up ordering too much. Don't think that just because restaurants offer three or more courses you have to sample them all—two should be sufficient, so don't be pressured into eating more than you want.

## 10 steps to a memorable meal out

1 Ignore any potato chips, nuts, or bread on the table. Occupy yourself by drinking water or a spicy tomato juice, rather than an aperitif (which stimulates the appetite and lures you into eating more than you need).

2 If you're offered bread with your main course—which you should really have only if you haven't ordered potatoes, rice, pasta, or any other starchy food—accept it only if it's fresh. If not, wave it away, because eating stale bread simply isn't worth the calories and sluggish effect on your body.

3 Do your body a favor and order relatively light dishes, like broiled meats, fish, or chicken, or those cooked in wine, rather than drenched in a thick sauce; pasta with a tomato sauce or risotto made with fresh stock.

4 Order salads and plenty of vegetable accompaniments. Ask for any oil, butter, or cream to be used sparingly in dressings, as these fats provide needless calories and mask the crisp flavors of the fresh ingredients.

5 When it comes to dessert, skipping pies and pastries will be easier on your digestive system and your waistline. Opt for fruit-based desserts like poached fruits and sorbets, rather than ice cream. Even better, round off your meal with a herbal infusion or decaffeinated coffee; and if you crave something sweet, have a piece of dark chocolate (which is high in antioxidants). Mmmm.

6 When traveling in Europe, you may be offered the option of cheese instead of (or in addition to!) dessert. If you opt for cheese, try to limit the damage. Cut the rind off a soft cheese to decrease its fat content, and enjoy your cheese with celery, fruit, or a whole-grain cracker, which will provide your body with some fiber to cushion its absorption of the fat and will help to fill you up.

7 Whether eating out or in, if the food isn't good, don't eat it. However, if this would cause offense, have only a small amount. Similarly, if you don't like what's on your plate or you've had enough, simply stop eating.

8 Be warned that a dessert wine, liqueur, port, or brandy can spoil your memories of an evening. These drinks have a high alcohol content that can irritate sensitive digestions, are loaded with calories, and can trigger blood-sugar swings that may keep you awake and leave you very hungover in the morning.

9 It's best to keep your alcohol intake down and to sip plenty of water throughout your meal, which, besides aiding digestion, will also cleanse your palate. What's more, because your taste buds will really register the flavor of each mouthful of food, you'll be satisfied with a smaller amount.

10 Never believe that because you've had only a small amount of alcohol it's safe to drive, because it isn't. Don't kid yourself that a cup of strong black coffee will sober you up, either. If you're driving, leave alcohol alone.

# bodyfoods solutions for eating on the move

However good our nutritional intentions, most of us tend to backslide when traveling. You only need to look at the food offered in fast-food restaurants and cafés, and on planes and trains, to understand why healthy eating on the move isn't easy. Having tried, over the years, to find good foods while in transit, I've come to the conclusion that the best way of maintaining your well-being on the move is to take your sustenance with you. I know: having to think of yet more things to pack before leaving home is tedious and time consuming; but believe me, investing a little time and effort will reward you with a more comfortable journey, so that you arrive raring to go.

## *keep well watered when on the go*

Traveling—especially in a plane, but also in any air-conditioned or heated vehicle—dehydrates the body, causing you to feel lethargic and headachy; and if you're flying, your fingers and feet swell. The first ally to enlist is water. You may think that the less water you drink, the less you'll retain, but the opposite, in fact, occurs. Drinking more water will help your body to balance its fluid system, particularly if you've been tucking into complimentary salty nibbles and nuts. (In any case, it's best to refuse salty snacks, as well as alcohol and sugary drinks like colas, all of which can trigger headaches and deplete energy levels.)

Try to drink a couple of small glasses of water every hour of your journey; or, if you're driving, regularly swig water from a small bottle (ideally stopping the car if you're the driver). I know that you will have to visit the restroom regularly, but you can limit the frequency by taking sips of water rather than swigging a lot at once. Walking to the restroom, or stopping at a service station, will help to keep you refreshed and focused. Indeed, studies now indicate that blood clots are common after sitting still, not only on long-haul flights, but on long car journeys, too, and that dehydration increases the risk of developing deep-vein thrombosis (DVT).

Because drinking too much tea and coffee dehydrates the body and unsettles the digestion, I'd advise skipping them and instead opting for herbal tea. If you're flying, stash a supply of herbal tea bags in your hand luggage, and ask the cabin crew to provide you with cups of hot water in which to infuse them. If you're driving or traveling on public transportation, procure some hot water from a service station or café or, cheaper still, fill a small vacuum flask with boiling water and take it with you. Although overdosing on coffee or tea may make you feel agitated and wobbly, which isn't safe when you're driving, if you're feeling tired and have to continue your journey, have the occasional cup to perk you up, but keep drinking plenty of water, too.

## my nutritious travel kit

- Water
- Herbal teas
- Fresh fruits: the most practical to eat on the move include grapes, tangerines or satsumas (oranges tend to squirt all over the place), small bananas, and apples, which you can slice and pack in a small plastic storage box
- Dried fruits, which contain fiber and slow-release sugar, are also high in potassium, a mineral that reduces fluid retention, so before you set off, I'd recommend stocking up with dried fruits, such as dates, figs, apricots, or mangoes (preferably without added sulfur dioxide, $SO_2$)
- Unsalted nuts, such as walnuts, almonds, and cashews
- Cold sliced meats, such as lean ham (but not fatty salami)
- Cheese cut into small chunks or the individually wrapped portions sold by supermarkets
- Swedish-style crisp breads and oatcakes make perfect partners for the cheese, and they are more easily digestible than bread
- Dips, such as bought or home-made guacamole or hummus, to team with crudités and hunks of hard cheese

On the following pages are some recipes for snacks that both travel well and taste great. (I suggest that you also look at the Energy-boosting Snacks on pages 58–9 for further inspiration.) And remember that it's best to keep all home-prepared food refrigerated for as long as possible before leaving home to minimize the risk of contamination by food-poisoning bacteria.

My final tips for when flying are, firstly, to stash some echinacea in your hand luggage to boost your immune system and help it resist the bacteria and viruses circulating around the cabin. (The recommended dose is either a 500mg capsule or tablet or 3/4–1 tsp. tincture dissolved in a small amount of water, taken three times a day.) Secondly, if you tend to suffer from stomach or bowel bloating, take some acidophilus pills (the recommended dose is about 20mg a day), preferably with a little yogurt or else some noncarbonated water.

If you still think it is too much bother to pack your own travel food, consider this: it's you, not the airline, train company, or highway service station, who has your body's best interests at heart. Look after your body, and you'll reap the dividends, unlike the passenger next to you, who is unenthusiastically munching his way through a plastic tray of tasteless food or a stodgy sandwich, courtesy of the airline or train company. So when packing your suitcase, remember that packing the right nutrients into your body will help you sail through your journey, wherever you may be headed.

# nutritious travel snacks

### SESAME AND POPPY SEED PITA STICKS (SERVES 4)

*A quick and easy way to make a tasty snack that can be dunked in one of your favorite dips.*

Heat the oven to 350°. Place 4 wholewheat pita breads on a baking tray. Heat in the oven for 1–2 minutes or until they bulge slightly. Split open each pita to leave two separate halves. Cut each half across the shortest width into 1-in. strips. Put 3 Tbs. olive oil into a large bowl and add seasoning. Toss the pita strips in the oil until thoroughly coated. In a small bowl, mix 2 Tbs. each sesame and poppy seeds. Sprinkle over the pita strips and toss together. Arrange the pita strips on a large baking sheet, and bake for 5–6 minutes or until lightly golden. Leave to cool.

### CIDER APPLE CAKE (MAKES A 7-IN. CAKE)

*This English cake is packed full of apples. Try to use a cider with a medium-sweet flavour.*

| | |
|---|---|
| 1 stick butter, softened | 1 tsp. mixed spice |
| scant $1/2$ cup granulated brown sugar | $1/2$ tsp. grated nutmeg |
| 2 eggs, beaten | $5/8$ cup plus 1 Tbs. hard cider |
| scant 2 cups, self-rising whole-grain flour | 1 large cooking apple, peeled and grated |

Heat the oven to 350°. Grease a 7-in. square cake pan and line the base with parchment paper. In a large bowl beat together the butter and sugar until light and fluffy, then gradually beat in the eggs. Gently fold in the flour, mixed spice, and nutmeg. Stir in the cider and apple. Spoon into the prepared pan, and bake in the oven for 40–45 minutes or until a toothpick inserted into the middle comes out clean. Leave to cool slightly, then turn out onto a wire rack to cool completely. Cut into squares before serving.

### BANANA PIZZA (SERVES 4)

*I know it sounds weird, but try it. If you're at home, serve it with some Greek-style yogurt as a dessert.*

Heat the oven to 425°. Empty 6 oz. package of pizza crust mix into a bowl and add 1 Tbs. confectioners' sugar. Stir in 1 generous Tbs. sunflower oil and enough warm water (about $5/8$ cup) to make a soft dough. Turn out onto a floured surface and knead for 5 minutes or until smooth. Roll out to a thin approximately 12-in. round, and transfer to a greased baking sheet. Put in a warm place for 10 minutes to rise. Peel 4 large bananas, slice into $1/2$-in. diagonals, and scatter over the pizza base. Sprinkle with the juice of 1 lemon and 2 Tbs. soft dark brown sugar. Bake in the oven for 10 minutes, then slip off the baking sheet directly onto the oven shelf and bake for another 10 minutes or until golden.

## WHITE CHOCOLATE CHIP COOKIES (MAKES 16)

*Homemade cookies are the best, especially when accompanied by ice-cold milk. Do not use commercial chocolate chips; chop up some chocolate from a bar, so you get real chunks.*

Heat the oven to 375°. In a food processor blend together 1 1/2 sticks softened butter, a scant 3/4 cup granulated brown sugar, and 1/2 tsp. vanilla extract, until light and creamy. Add 3/4 cup flour and 3/4 cup, rounded, finely milled whole-grain self-rising flour. Process again until thoroughly mixed together. Turn the mixture out into a large bowl and fold in 3/4 cup, rounded, roughly chopped white chocolate. Shape the mixture into 16 even-sized balls, then flatten them slightly. Place them on a baking sheet, leaving enough room for them to spread while baking. Bake for 15 minutes or until golden. Allow to cool slightly before transfering to a wire rack to cool completely.

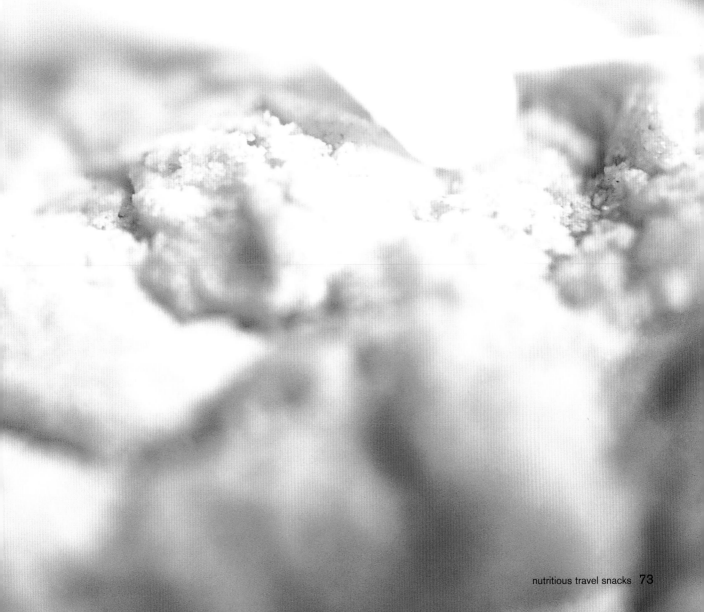

# comforting treats

## CELERY STALKS STUFFED WITH GOAT CHEESE AND CHIVES (SERVES 2)

*These are not only good comfort nibbles but also delicious as canapés to have with drinks.*

Scrub clean 2 or 3 green, crunchy celery stalks and cut off the tough ends. Slice the stalks into 2-in. chunks and set them to one side. In small bowl, mix 4½ oz. soft, young goat cheese with ½ tsp. chopped fresh chives, and season with freshly ground black pepper. Dollop a little of the cheese mixture onto the concave side of each celery chunk, and serve at once.

## CRUNCHY PEANUT AND COLESLAW OPEN SANDWICH (SERVES 2)

*A very quick and healthful alternative to perk up a peanut butter sandwich. If you cannot find a coleslaw salad mix, just use a little grated carrot, cabbage, and onion.*

Spread 1 Tbs. peanut butter per slice over 4 slices of wholewheat bread. Top with a handful of ready-to-use coleslaw salad mix. Drizzle a little olive oil and a squeeze of lemon juice on top. Now add 1 Tbs. roughly chopped mint and a handful of raisins, then season well. Serve immediately.

## VANILLA HONEYED YOGURT (SERVES 4)

*Creamy natural yogurt is perfectly sweetened with honey and vanilla. Why not serve it with a few mixed summer berries?.*

Start by roughly chopping a scant 3/4 cup hazelnuts, and carefully toast under a high broiler for 3–4 minutes or until lightly golden. Leave to cool. Spoon 2 cups natural bio yogurt into a bowl, and stir in 1 tsp. vanilla extract and 3 Tbs. clear honey. Mix well. When ready to serve, spoon the yogurt into glass dishes and sprinkle with the toasted hazelnuts.

## RAISINS WITH ROASTED SEEDS

Place ¼ cup sunflower seeds on a baking tray and pop them under a hot broiler for a couple of minutes to turn them golden brown (watch carefully to make sure they don't burn). Allow them to cool, and then mix with ½ cup, rounded, organic raisins, ¼ cup sesame seeds, and 3 Tbs. flaxseeds.

## NIGEL SLATER'S CHOCOLATE ICE CREAM (SERVES 4)

*This recipe, from the well-known British cookery writer, Nigel Slater, was the first ice cream I made using my ice-cream maker. It's deliciously indulgent, but low in sugar, and I've used decaffeinated coffee to keep the caffeine intake down.*

**7 oz. dark chocolate (with minimum 70% cocoa solids)**

**1 freshly made decaffeinated espresso coffee**

**1 3/4 cups ready-made custard sauce**

**1 cup plus 1 Tbs. heavy cream**

Break the chocolate into pieces and place in the top of a double boiler. Add the espresso coffee. Place the bowl over a pan of boiling water, being careful not to allow the bottom of the bowl to touch the water. Melt the chocolate, then remove from the heat. Meanwhile, in a jug, mix the custard and the cream together. Allow the chocolate to cool for a couple of minutes, before adding a little of the custard mixture to the chocolate bowl and mixing thoroughly to form a smooth, thick chocolate custard. Then add the remaining creamy mixture, stirring well before placing inside the ice-cream maker. In roughly 20 minutes you'll have the most delicious chocolaty dessert you could ever imagine.

If you can't find ready-made custard sauce, or crème anglaise, follow the recipe for custard on page 122, increasing the quantities to 1 5/8 cups milk, a rounded Tbs. of sugar, and 2 large eggs.

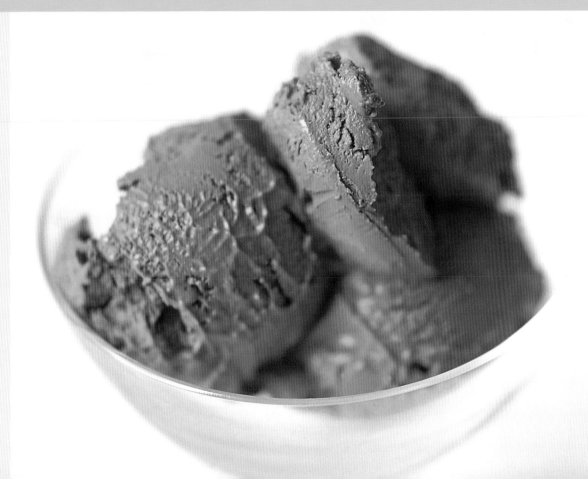

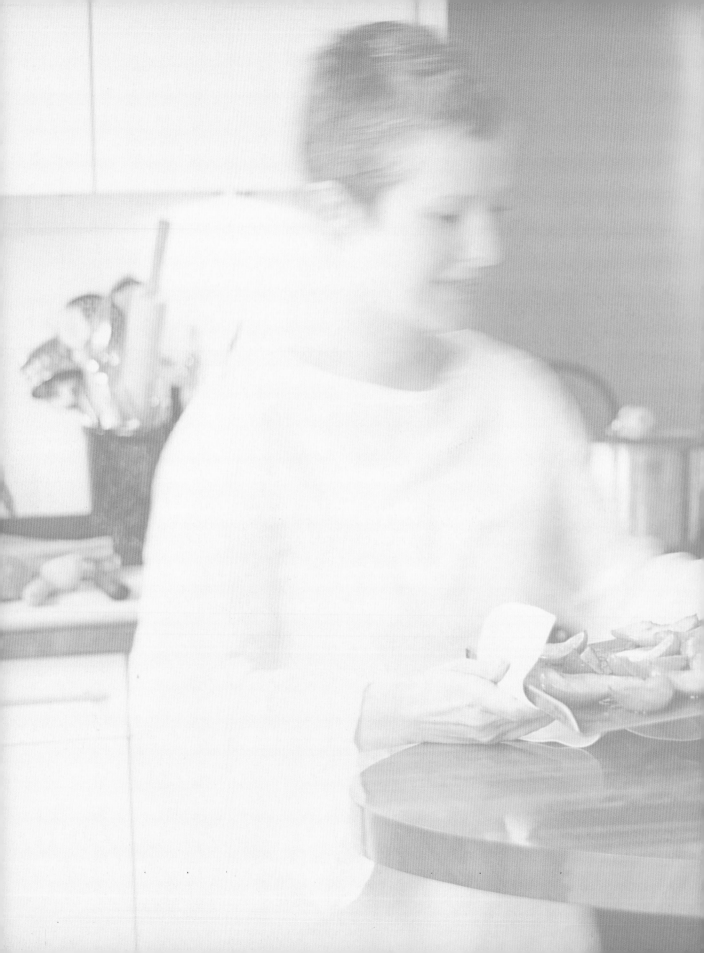

# bodyfoods
# therapies

It can be tempting to pop a pill or reach for a medicine when your body complains under the strain of a busy life. Although it's hard to believe, the food and drink you consume have a much better chance of providing you with an efficient healer. The solutions are simple, straightforward, and not rocket science involving new theories that need brain space to work through. I've done the hard work, so that you can eat and drink to soothe the physical and emotional effects of being overly stretched.

# beating headaches and migraines

The bane of a busy life, headaches always come when we have least time to cope with them. They range from hangover-related ones through cluster headaches to chronic migraines. Although the types are physiologically different, nutritionists treat them in a similar way, first asking sufferers to keep a food-and-mood diary for two weeks, listing everything they eat and drink, as well as how they feel and any symptoms. This often reveals a link between nutrition and the incidence of headaches and migraines, one of the strongest being eating tyramine-rich foods (including herrings, sharp cheeses, peanuts and peanut butter, chocolate, variety meats, cured sausages, and sauerkraut) and drinking alcohol, closely followed by eating foods that contain monosodium glutamate (MSG or E621), especially processed products and Chinese food.

Other common triggers, especially when you're hungry or stressed, include caffeine, be it coffee, tea, cola, or chocolate. Totting up ten cups of coffee during the day, and then having another before a meeting, can spell disaster. I'd generally recommend steering clear of caffeine-containing drinks and instead having either a glass of room-temperature water or a mug of warm herbal tea (temperature's important because extremes can also trigger headaches). Strangely enough, a single dose of caffeine can occasionally alleviate a headache, and if you've found that this sometimes works for you, it's best to take your "medicine" in the form of a cup of tea, which is gentler on both head and body. This relieving effect is more pronounced in caffeine addicts, which doesn't mean that being addicted to caffeine is a good thing. Indeed, you'll feel so much better if you wean yourself off it; but be warned that the first forty-eight hours may be blighted by a caffeine-withdrawal headache—but then you're used to that.

Drinking alcohol on an empty stomach, or when you're dehydrated, exhausted, or stressed, can also saddle you with an almighty headache or migraine the next day. Champagne and red wine, which are rich in phenolic compounds, are the worst offenders, followed by white wine, which is very acidic. You probably already know which alcoholic drink affects your head the worst, so avoid it and always down lots of water before, during, and after drinking alcohol. If, despite these precautions, you still wake up with a hangover headache, try a cup of detoxifying dandelion tea (see pages 82–3 for other hangover-targeting tips).

If you're prone to headaches and migraines, one of the worst things you can do is eat very sweet foods on an empty stomach, because this swiftly brings about headache-inducing blood-sugar changes. Some of the sufferers I treat wonder if they're suffering from hypoglycemia (an abnormally low blood-sugar level) because they feel lousy when they're hungry and better after they've eaten, but they are then flummoxed when their blood-sugar level is measured and found to be normal. The simple explanation is that your blood-sugar level may occasionally either drop a little too low or drop (or rise) too quickly, all of which can trigger headaches and migraines. If any of these scenarios sound familiar, I'd advise avoiding sweet foods as far as possible and incorporating more whole grains (see pages 40–43) into your diet. We all give in to our cravings for sweet treats from time to time, but the secret lies in picking the ones that won't make your head pound, such as a cake made with whole-grain flour.

Indeed, eating high-fiber foods, such as whole grains and fresh vegetables and fruits, may be of significant help to your poor head (but treat citrus fruits with caution because they can cause headaches and migraines). If, however, you are hit by a headache after eating whole-grain bread and cereals, consult your doctor or dietician, because you may have an allergy or intolerance to gluten. Snacking on fresh or dried fruits—preferably organic—and having frequent small meals will keep your blood-sugar level steady, and consequently your head. Another advantage is that it will keep your digestive system functioning smoothly, thereby averting constipation-related headaches, which can also be fended off by boosting your fiber intake and steadily drinking your way through a daily 5 pints of water.

Finally, some recent research suggests that increasing your intake of oily fish may reduce the incidence of headaches and migraines, so try having fresh tuna, salmon, sardines, or mackerel a couple of times a week. An alternative for non-fish eaters (but not strict vegetarians) is to take a fish-oil supplement.

## checklist of headache causes and solutions

Are you dehydrated? Dehydration commonly brings on both a headache and poor concentration, so fend them off by drinking 5 pints of water each day.

Are you constipated? Constipation also causes headaches, so ward it off by drinking plenty of water and eating lots of fiber-packed fresh and dried fruits, seeds (try my delicious Raisins with Roasted Seeds on page 74) and vegetables.

Have you been drinking too much alcohol and drinks containing caffeine? In addition to alcohol, tea, coffee, chocolate, and cola are all particularly draining beverages, so have them in moderation.

When was the last time you ate a proper meal? If it was many hours ago, your blood-sugar level may be too low and your head may be protesting. Snacking between meals is the best way to maintain a good supply of blood sugar to the brain, and the best snacks are fresh or dried fruits or whole-grain cookies.

Did you drink orange juice on an empty stomach first thing this morning? Eating too many citrus fruits can encourage your body to absorb headache-inducing copper irons, so you'd be better off opting for less acidic fruits, such as apples, mangoes, pineapples, and bananas.

Did you skip breakfast? An empty stomach finds it hard to feed an active brain, so eating something, however little, in the morning will increase your concentration and ward off a headache. Try to breakfast on a slow-release whole grain (toast or cereal) or a smoothie (see page 81).

# bodyfoods solutions for headaches and migraines

### MY FAVORITE OATCAKES (MAKES 8)

*This is my own sweet variation on a traditional Scottish recipe.*

3/4 cup all-purpose flour

1/4 tsp. baking soda

scant 1/2 cup brown crystal sugar

scant 1 cup rolled oats

3/4 stick butter

1 Tbs. corn syrup

scant 1/4 cup pumpkin seeds

Heat the oven to 325°. Sift the flour and baking soda into a bowl. Add the sugar and oats and mix well. In a saucepan, melt the butter with the corn syrup over a low heat (taking care not to let it boil), and then pour the liquid over the oat mixture, stirring with a wooden spoon. When it is cool enough to handle, form the mixture into a ball on a floured surface. Roll out to a thickness of about 1 in. and cut it into rounds. Place the rounds on a lightly oiled baking sheet and sprinkle with the pumpkin seeds. Bake in the oven for 15 minutes or until golden brown. Place on a wire rack to cool.

### EASY TOMATO AND BASIL PASTA SAUCE (SERVES 8)

*Not only is this pasta sauce incredibly easy to make; it can be kept in the fridge to enjoy the next day (in which case, lift the flavors by sprinkling it with a dash of olive oil once you've added the cooked pasta to the sauce).*

3 cups small fresh basil leaves

3 1/2 cups canned Italian plum tomatoes,
    drained, deseeded, and roughly chopped

12 garlic cloves, peeled and minced

1/2 cup olive oil

sea salt and freshly ground black pepper

Remove and discard the stalks from the basil leaves, then rinse in cold water. Pat dry with paper towels and chop roughly. Place the tomatoes in a large saucepan. Set aside 1 Tbs. of the basil leaves and add the remainder to the pan, along with the garlic and olive oil. Cook over a medium heat for about 30 minutes, stirring often to prevent the mixture from sticking to the pan. Season with some sea salt and plenty of freshly ground black pepper. Throw in the reserved basil and stir.

## BANANA AND VANILLA SMOOTHIE (SERVES 1)

*This non-acidic, pure-fruit smoothie is rich in slow-release sugars.*

Place 6 oz. organic vanilla yogurt and 2 ripe (but not mushy) bananas in a blender. Process until smooth. Depending on the desired thickness, add a dash of milk. Serve immediately.

## APRICOT AND ALMOND SCONES (MAKES 12)

*Scones (a British relative of the American biscuit) are fantastic to bake, as most of the time you have the ingredients on hand and they take no time at all to make. Your kitchen will smell heavenly.*

scant 1/4 cup whole-grain pastry flour

baking powder

1/2 cup ground almonds

1/2 stick butter, softened

2 Tbs. granulated brown sugar

pinch of salt

2 tsp. almond extract

1/2 cup, rounded ready-to-eat dried apricots,
 finely chopped

5/8 cup milk

Heat the oven to 425°. Place the flour and almonds in a large bowl, and rub in the butter. Stir in the sugar, salt, almond extract and apricots. Make a well in the center of the mix, and pour in enough milk to bring the mixture to a dough. Turn out onto a floured surface and knead lightly until smooth. Roll out to a thickness of 1-in., then, using a 2-in. round pastry cutter, cut out 12 scones. Lay them, evenly spaced, on a greased baking sheet, and brush with a little milk. Bake in the oven for 10–12 minutes or until risen and lightly golden.

## *herbal first aid for headaches and migraines*

If you're desperate for immediate relief, one of the best first-aid measures is to massage a few drops of lavender essential oil into your temples. Feverfew, skullcap, and rosemary, which can be administered in various ways, are also good herbal remedies, as is mint tea, especially when you suspect that something you've eaten has given you a headache or migraine. I also find vervain tea an effective reliever of nervous and stress-related headaches, but don't take it if you're pregnant. At the first sign of a migraine, take 10 drops of feverfew in water, unless you're pregnant. If the migraine has already kicked in, infuse 1 heaped tsp. skullcap in 1 cup warm water (you can take up to 4 cups a day). Lime helps to relieve tension headaches, so try adding 1 heaped tsp. lime juice to 1 cup warm water and drinking up to 5 cups a day.

# coping with jet lag and hangovers

Travel is becoming more and more part of our routine as cheap flights and world business pressures kick in. Property prices and pollution also drive us out of the cities. But traveling, forcing us to commute to work affects our bodies in numerous ways—from feeling acidic in the gut, to your head appearing to be in a different place from your body. Excess drinking can feel like a short-term fix for escaping the pressure of life, but it's a quick ticket to hangover hell and a body that's foggy, tired, and fed up with being on the treadmill.

The following tips will help you to minimize the symptoms of hangovers and jet lag.

## tips to avoid jet lag and travel sickness

- If you know that you're likely to suffer from travel sickness, enlist the aid of ginger. Sipping a cup of ginger tea (see page 13), sucking a little gingerroot or some ginger lozenges, or swallowing a ginger capsule (you can safely take 500mg three times a day) will all help to alleviate nausea.
- Sprinkling a few drops of lavender or camomile essential oil on a cotton handkerchief or over your pillow on the flight can encourage you to rest and sleep.
- Many people believe that staying awake for as long as possible is the best cure for jet lag once you've arrived in a different time zone. However, I find that having a bath to which I've added a few drops of grapefruit and lavender essential oil, and then going to bed, work wonders.
- Once you've arrived at your destination, try to eat light foods rather than tucking into the heavy, rich, sauce-based dishes that challenge the gut, especially if you're expecting it to deal with a large meal when it would normally receive breakfast. Similarly, if you've arrived in a country that has a spicy cuisine, such as Thailand or India, your digestive system may struggle with its chili- and spice-laden dishes, so start off with as bland a local delicacy as possible—for example, a simple dhal in India.
- If you're feeling generally jumpy and unsettled, remember that pasta, rice, and other starchy foods are good for settling the stomach and promoting sleep.
- Protein-rich foods like eggs and meat, as well as vegetables and fruits, can stimulate a sluggish body, making them good choices if you're trying to energize a body that thinks it should still be sleeping.
- Keep your energy levels constant by having small meals often and snacking on healthful tidbits like fruits and unsalted nuts.
- It's best to avoid alcohol and to limit your caffeine intake to the occasional milky coffee or cup of tea—that is, unless your body is about to give up on you and you need to jolt it into action, in which case an espresso may do the trick.

## 8 ways to handle hangover hell

1 Take milk thistle to encourage your liver to detoxify itself. Make a decoction using 1 Tbs. dandelion root to 1³/₄ pints water, and take it in small quantities, at frequent intervals, throughout the day.

2 Drink lots of water or herbal tea (see pages 12–13). Dandelion, mint, and fennel are particularly good system cleansers, but if you don't have one of these on hand, any herbal infusion will rehydrate your body, as, of course, will water. If you dislike the taste of plain water, add a little fruit juice—ideally one that is high in fruit, but low in sugar, and not a very sweet syrup, whose effect will be to unsettle your blood-sugar level (which the alcohol has depressed), making you feel worse. Take small sips steadily.

3 Avoid coffee, particularly espresso, as its caffeine content can prompt your body to lose even more water, which, because a hangover is primarily caused by dehydration, is the last thing you need. Caffeine can also make you feel wired and jittery, compounding your hangover symptoms. Although tea contains caffeine, too, as do cola and chocolate, if it is weak, a couple of cups can act as a good restorative, especially if you add milk; but switch to non-caffeine-containing fluids thereafter.

4 Try to eat something, however small, as soon as you can stand the thought. Some people swear by a high-protein breakfast or brunch of eggs and bacon. This will certainly help to restore your blood-sugar level, and hence strength, to normal; so if you can manage it, great.

5 If you can't face a cooked breakfast, some wholewheat toast or cereal, or, failing that, a banana, an oatmeal cookie, a small tub of yogurt, or a smoothie made with fruits that aren't too acidic, such as mangoes, bananas, papayas or melon, will return your blood-sugar level to the comfort zone.

6 Steer well clear of fatty foods, such as the croissants and pastries sold by breakfast bars, which can be too hard for a hungover gut to digest. Not only that, syrupy pastries can cause a blood-sugar high, followed by a sudden crash, thereby exacerbating your symptoms and leaving you feeling bloated and liverish. This is why your cooked breakfast should comprise lean, grilled bacon and poached eggs, rather than fatty sausages and scrambled eggs drenched in butter, and why your cereal should be of the whole-grain, fruit-and-fiber type, not a sugary one.

7 If you're on the run, give candy bars a wide berth, too—you're far better off buying a savory oat cracker or a slice of toast from a café, while a Canadian bacon sandwich made with whole-wheat bread may be just the thing to restore your *joie de vivre*.

8 Forget another drink—it will only prolong your hangover and, indeed, make it ten times worse.

# tackling sleep problems and deficiency

Lack of sleep can be incredibly debilitating. If you don't get enough hours of slumber (and I, for one, need eight), you wake up feeling shattered, can't rise to the demands of the day, and go to bed again feeling thoroughly stressed, which in turn prevents you from sleeping well and sets up a vicious cycle.

Sleep triggers your body to release growth hormone, which increases the absorption of nutrients by cells, encourages the growth and repair of bone and muscle, and stimulates the immune system. Under the influence of growth hormone, cells are most active and divide the most when you're asleep; sleep deprivation soon shows in your skin, as its cells need to be constantly replaced to keep you looking fresh and healthy.

Your health and appearance are also influenced by the type of sleep you get. As most cell renewal occurs during deep sleep, your skin, for example, soon loses its clarity and bloom if this stage of sleep is disturbed. When our bodies have an increased need for growth—when we're young or pregnant, for instance—the amount of both deep sleep and growth hormone increases (so don't chastise your teenagers for sleeping too much—their bodies are getting on with the business of growing!).

## sweet dreams

A comforting glass of cold milk helps me to sleep—perhaps because my father always brought me a bedtime glass of milk when I was a child—but, in fact, some interesting new research into milk has shown that it can aid slumber. Night milk (stocked by some supermarkets) is so called because it is from cows milked at night. It contains especially high levels of melatonin, a hormone reputed to offer many beneficial properties, including those that delay the aging process, ward off diseases, and prolong life. All types of milk provide your body with tryptophan and milk sugars, both of which encourage the brain to produce the hormone serotonin, which, because it makes you feel contented, is a natural aid to sleep. Milk also contains magnesium, another sleep-promoter. If you don't like milk, green vegetables, nuts, and whole grains are rich in this nutrient, too. However, it's best not to add cocoa powder or chocolate to milk—or at least not a lot of it—because the caffeine these substances contain (as do tea, coffee and cola) acts as a stimulant.

I sometimes like to have a glass of wine to help me unwind, but drinking too much is likely to disturb my sleep and leave me feeling weary. Excessive amounts of alcohol (especially when drunk on an empty stomach before crawling into bed) can cause your blood-sugar level to drop and your body to become dehydrated. If you're tempted to have a drink, make it a small one and team it with food (see pages 26–7 and 78), even if it's a quickly put together tapas plate with hot toast or some roasted organic nuts.

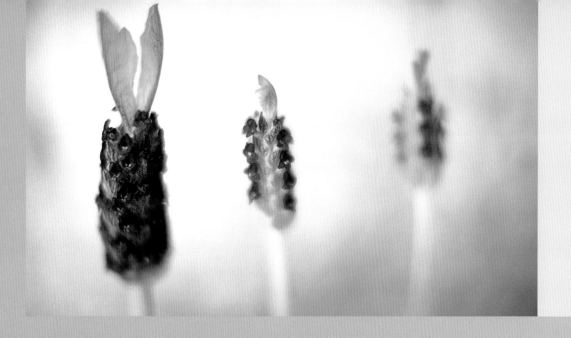

The types of food that you eat can have an impact on how you sleep, too. Very sweet foods, such as cookies and candy, are best avoided because they can cause your blood-sugar level to rise, making you feel hyperactive. Cheese and meat, on the other hand, may give you bad dreams, or even nightmares, while an evening meal that consists primarily of protein-rich foods, including again meat, chicken, or fish, may energize you—which is great if you have sex in mind, because not only is an orgasm a superb sleep trigger but sex also stimulates a burst of growth hormone, but may otherwise prevent you from dropping off.

By contrast, the best foods with which to induce a soporific state are starchy carbohydrates, including potatoes, pasta, and rice. These foods stimulate the brain to produce serotonin, which is why I find a big bowl of pasta one of the best sleep inducers. If you arrive home and don't have the time or energy to cook, a bowl of milky hot cereal may have a similar effect (try my Cardamom Rice Milk Porridge on page 42).

Although it's best to have something to eat before retiring for the night, try not to eat too late, or too much, because having a full stomach can lead to indigestion. Many experts advise not eating after 6 P.M.; but this is easier said than done if, like myself, you don't finish work until long after that and consequently end up having dinner at 8 P.M. or later. To avert the hunger pangs that will tempt you to overeat at such a late hour, have a late-afternoon snack (see pages 58–9) to tide you over until you've at last got the time to have a small, starchy evening meal (see pages 60–65).

## herbal first aid for sleep problems

Herbal teas are better options than either caffeine-containing or alcoholic nightcaps; camomile, lemon balm, passion flower, and valerian, in particular, can lull you into a deep, refreshing sleep. You may also find that adding a few drops of clary sage, sandalwood, or marjoram essential oil to your bath and sprinkling a little lavender essential oil over your pillow soon sends you floating off toward the Land of Nod.

# coping with chronic fatigue

Most of us can cope with the occasional day of feeling tired—and acute fatigue can usually be resolved by a few good nights' sleep—but chronic fatigue can be one of the most debilitating conditions to battle against, especially when you're leading a busy life.

Waking up to yet another day of being so exhausted you feel as though you haven't slept for weeks can raise serious doubts about whether you can make it through the coming hours. At its worst, chronic fatigue can leave you living under a cloud of anxiety, feeling so uncertain about your body's ability to stand up to the demands of the day that you may end up having panic attacks. And if you're used to being a high achiever, finding that your body is no longer able to keep up with your punishing schedule can lead to depression.

Chronic fatigue can be a symptom of many underlying conditions, including anemia, blood-sugar imbalance, an underactive thyroid gland (see pages 112–15), depression, and chronic fatigue syndrome (CFS), so if you're constantly exhausted, ask your doctor for a blood test. More typically, however, there is no medical explanation, except, perhaps, a virus, which can cause some sufferers to become so exhausted that they are unable to stir from their beds, sometime also being stricken by symptoms like swollen glands in the throat, armpits, and groin, tonsillitis, aching muscles, fever, loss of appetite, depression, and weakness.

If you've contracted a viral infection that makes you feel chronically tired, there's a danger that you won't be able to muster either the inclination or the energy to eat properly, thus depriving your body of the energizing nutrients that it's crying out for. If this continues, your weakened immune system may start losing the battle against the virus, which may consequently develop into a longer-term and more incapacitating condition like CFS, which can follow in the wake of mononucleosis, itself caused by the Epstein-Barr virus.

## take time out

When you're suffering from chronic fatigue inflicted by a viral illness, it's definitely not a case of business as usual. It's vital that you bow out of the rat race for a while, and rest as much as possible, to conserve your precious energy for such essential tasks as eating nutritiously. Try, however, to set yourself small targets and to maintain your normal sleeping routine, rather than getting into the habit of spending your days in bed. The less purpose or structure there is to your life, the more likely it will be that you'll drift into a depressive type of existence, so that the less you do, the less you'll feel like doing. It's far better to follow an early-to-bed regime, to set the alarm clock, and, when you get up, to take some gentle exercise in the fresh air to encourage energizing oxygen to circulate around your body. Practicing some stress-busting exercises (see pages 147, 148, and 150) may also boost your energy levels.

Most importantly, keep eating nutritious foods, because the more healthful nutrients your body receives, the quicker it will recover. If you really can't face preparing a meal, then a smoothie, chopped banana, a bowl of fresh soup from the deli counter, some scrambled eggs, an omelet, or a baked potato is better than nothing (see Favorite Combinations for Late Meals in 10 Minutes on page 63 for more ideas). If friends or relatives have rallied to your bedside, ask one of them to make you a big pan of my Easy Tomato and Basil Pasta Sauce (see page 80), which is packed with the virus-fighting antioxidants vitamins A and E and lycopene. Divide it among small containers to freeze or refrigerate, which gives you lots of helpings to team with boiled dried pasta (which contains energizing starches) and protein-rich Parmesan cheese.

Eat as many fresh vegetables, salads, and fruits as you can manage, to reap the much-needed, immune-system-boosting benefits of the vitamin C that they provide. Mix a few summer berries, chopped small fruits or orange segments with some natural yogurt or milk (both of which contain vitamin B, another ally of the immune system), or blend them into a smoothie. (For an intense hit of nutrients, try my Blueberry, Banana, and Orange Vitamin-C Boosting Smoothie on page 15.) You can also derive B vitamins from whole grains, brown rice, cheese, eggs, fish, dried fruits (which make sustaining snacks), bananas, spinach, and broccoli.

On the subject of B vitamins, supplements may be just the tonic you need in a nutritional emergency, so I'd therefore advise taking a vitamin B-complex supplement, a vitamin C supplement (1,000mg each morning), and some Siberian ginseng (500mg a day for six weeks), as well as giving your immune system another helping hand in the form of echinacea (500mg three times a day for about a month). A vitamin $B_{12}$ injection administered by your doctor may also perk you up.

Research suggests that essential fatty acids aid the body's recovery from debilitating viruses, so if you can face it, focus on eating oily fish, such as fresh tuna, salmon, mackerel, sardines, and trout. If oily fish is out of the question, try to have some protein-rich foods, including chicken, eggs, cheese, and legumes (like baked beans on toast), and the payback will be more energy, a stronger immune system, and a healthy dose of zinc, another enemy of viral infections.

My final advice is to avoid alcohol and caffeine, which undermine your energy levels in the long term (see pages 24–7). Instead drink at least 2.5 litres/4 pints water a day (see page 12–13). It is said that 600ml/1 pint of water equates to 20 per cent of extra energy, and I certainly find that I feel significantly tired and low when I haven't drunk enough water, but then perk up astoundingly quickly as soon as I've rehydrated my body. Not only do they provide water, but herbal teas like lemon verbena (see page 13) have the power to nurture a burned-out body.

# bodyfoods solutions for chronic fatigue

## MUNG AND FAVA BEAN DHAL (SERVES 4–6)

6 oz. yellow split mung beans (moong dal),
   picked over, cleaned, and washed

1 medium-sized onion, finely chopped

1¹/₂ Tbs. grated fresh gingerroot

2 tsp. minced garlic

¹/₂ tsp. turmeric

2 medium-sized potatoes,
   peeled and quartered

14 oz. fava beans, fresh or frozen

1 tsp. sea salt

5 large handfuls fresh spinach leaves,
   thoroughly washed with stalks removed

2 tsp. lemon juice

3 Tbs. cilantro leaves, chopped

*For the tadka*

2 Tbs. light vegetable oil

1 tsp. cumin seeds

1 green chili

sea salt and freshly ground black pepper

Put the mung beans in a deep pot with the onion, ginger, garlic, and 3 cups water. Add the turmeric and bring to the boil. Reduce heat, and simmer, partially covered, for 15 minutes or until the mung beans are cooked, but are still very firm. Add the potatoes, fava beans, salt, and 2 cups water. Cook for another 15 minutes or until the potato is tender and the beans are thoroughly cooked. Three minutes from the end of cooking, add the spinach leaves and stir to soften. To finish and bring out the flavors, make the tadka by heating the vegetable oil over a high heat in a skillet. When very hot, add the cumin seeds, and fry for about 15 seconds, until dark brown. Add the chili, stir for a moment, and immediately pour the contents of the frying pan into the stew. Add the lemon juice and the cilantro. Stir well to mix. Check the seasoning, then transfer the dhal to a heated serving dish.

## BROILED CINNAMON PAPAYA (SERVES 2)

*When buying a papaya, sniff it, rather than squeezing it; and if your nose detects a highly perfumed scent, this is a sure sign that the fruit is ripe and ready to eat.*

Heat the broiler to medium. Cut 1 large papaya in half, from its stem to its base. Remove and discard all of the brown seeds and stringy bits, and peel off the skin. Slice the papaya lengthwise into long strips. Arrange the papaya strips on a lightly oiled baking tray, and dust them with cinnamon. Place the baking tray under the broiler for 1–2 minutes. Serve immediately with some creamy vanilla ice cream or yogurt and a sprinkling of toasted coconut.

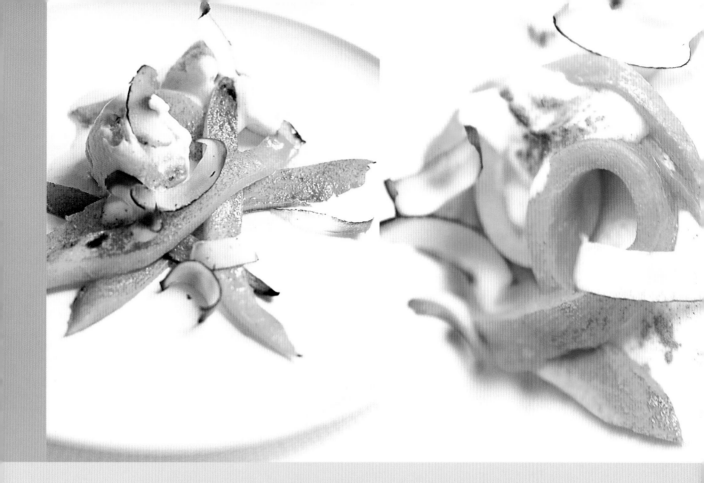

## FIG AND DATE COUSCOUS (SERVES 4)

*I love couscous because it's satisfying, but doesn't seem to cause an energy dip after eating it.*
*It's also very quick to make.*

1 1/4 cups couscous

3/8 cup figs, roughly chopped

3/8 cup Medjool dates, stoned and
  roughly chopped

5/8 cup dried apricots, roughly chopped

1/2 cup shelled pistachio nuts

scant 1/4 cup walnuts, chopped

lemon juice

small knob unsalted butter

Heat the oven to 350°. Place the couscous in a bowl, pour in an equal volume of cold water, and cover.
Stir occasionally until the grains have absorbed the water, which should take about 10–15 minutes.
Rub the couscous grains to break down any lumps. Now add the figs, dates, apricots, pistachio nuts, and
walnuts. Mix thoroughly, transfer to a shallow ovenproof dish, covering it with aluminum foil and sealing
the edges well to prevent the couscous from drying out. Bake in the oven for 20 minutes. Remove from
the oven, discard the foil, and then add a dash of lemon juice and a small knob of unsalted butter, fluffing
the couscous with a fork. Season to taste with a little sea salt and plenty of freshly ground black pepper.
Serve at once.

# combating colds, flu, and sinusitis

You've woken up with a cold and are desperate to clear your stuffy head and soothe your sore throat. Yet, because you caught the cold as a result of your immune system being weakened, you need not only to alleviate your symptoms but also to build up your body's defenses. The trouble with over-the-counter remedies is that although they can relieve the symptoms of cold, flu, and sinusitis, they do nothing for your immune system, leaving you vulnerable to the myriad other bugs flying around. And because colds spread like wildfire in air-conditioned and closed environments, it's advisable to focus on strengthening your immune system as soon as you, or anyone around you, succumbs to the sniffles.

You may not be able to ward off a cold forever, but a number of remedies will at least help you to feel better and function more efficiently. To begin with, try adding a few drops of eucalyptus or thyme essential oil (both powerful decongestants) to a bowl of boiling water, covering your head with a towel, leaning over the bowl, and then breathing in deeply as the water cools. A steam inhalation like this, both in the morning and at night, can really help to relieve sinus pain and congestion and sharpen a fuzzy brain. Enlisting the aid of another herbal remedy, echinacea (take 500mg three times a day for a few weeks), will also boost your immune system, helping both to banish and to fend off colds and flu.

## build your defenses

The main nutrients to boost when you've been struck down with a cold or flu, or are worried that you soon will be, are vitamin C and zinc, both of which support the immune system. The received wisdom that it's necessary to start taking very high doses of vitamin C supplements is not supported by scientific evidence, however; indeed, doing so can cause bloating, stomach disorders, and even more serious problems, such as kidney conditions. You're better off eating and drinking plenty of fresh, vitamin C-rich foods (see page 14), particularly citrus juices (preferably those that are as fresh as possible, rather than ones whose use-by dates are months away because they contain added sugar). Similarly, there is little evidence to support the benefits of taking zinc in supplement form, so you're best to focus on eating such zinc-rich foods as whole grains, nuts, seeds, and lean proteins like chicken and eggs.

There is, however, one instance when I'd recommend resorting to supplements, and that is if your cold or flu has robbed you of your appetite, in which case take a daily dose of 500mg vitamin C and 15mg zinc, along with echinacea (see above for the recommended dosage) and a garlic-oil capsule. If you're a smoker, try to quit, even if it's only temporarily, because not only does smoking exacerbate breathing problems, it reduces your body's vitamin C levels, too.

It's vital to keep up your fluid intake by constantly drinking water and soothing teas made with body-boosting herbs (see page 13) but avoiding caffeine-containing drinks and alcohol. A lemon and natural honey drink is one of my favorites when I'm laid low with a cold, because the lemon provides vitamin C and the honey both soothes a scratchy throat and has natural antibacterial, antiviral and antiseptic qualities (especially if it's a variety that contains UMF factor, such as Manuka). Because heat destroys honey's active properties, swallow 2 tsp. natural honey a couple of times a day, too. If this doesn't appeal, try mixing it with a little yogurt.

Garlic is another natural remedy with potent antiseptic and decongestant qualities, which is why I'd advise using plenty in your cooking, including it raw in salads and taking a garlic-oil supplement. Try my homemade hot-drink remedy (see below), too; but because it will make your breath smell a little overpowering, maybe it's best taken at bedtime! Ginger and chili are other good immune-system-boosters, so think along the lines of tea made with fresh gingerroot and stir-fries containing ginger and a little fresh chili.

Although some people claim that consuming dairy products increases mucus production, this has never been scientifically proven. However, if you notice this effect after drinking milk or eating cheese, yogurt, or butter, it may be worth decreasing your intake of these foods. If you do so, you'll need to ensure that your calcium status (see pages 36–9) isn't compromised by eating nondairy sources of this vital mineral, such as green, leafy vegetables, small-boned fish like sardines, dried fruits, seeds, and calcium-enriched soy products.

Besides taking these first-aid measures, getting as much rest as you can and trying to decrease your stress levels will speed your recovery. My mother's remedy for colds and fevers is a hot drink, a hot bath, followed by a hot bed—a combination that will raise your body temperature enough to sweat the bug out of your system. You could warm your bed with either a hot-water bottle or a hot bedfellow—regular sex having been shown to increase levels of IgA (a cold and flu antibody found in saliva) by up to 30 percent!

Once you're feeling up to exercising, don't overdo it while you're recuperating. You may think that a good workout will brush away the cobwebs—and, indeed, it may—but the downside of intensive exercise is that it suppresses the immune system, making the mouth and throat areas especially vulnerable to infection, which is why athletes are prone to infections of the upper respiratory tract. So by all means take a gentle stroll in the fresh air, but don't exercise too much when you have a fever or are feeling under par.

## *herbal first aid for colds*

- To make a potent cold remedy, crush a medium-sized garlic clove with a similar-sized piece of gingerroot. Mix with the juice of 1 lemon and 1 tsp. honey. Add warm water. Drink up to 3 cups a day.
- If you can't stand garlic, mix the juice of 1 lemon with 1 tsp. honey and 1/2 tsp. cinnamon powder.
- If you have nasal congestion, make an infusion by mixing thyme and boneset (1/2 tsp. each) with a cup of water, and drink 3–4 cups a day.

# bodyfoods solutions for colds and flu

### SALSA VERDE (SERVES 6–8)

*Your taste buds can need a real kick when you have a cold or flu—so try these salsas for size! If you prefer, you could use lemon juice instead of white wine vinegar. Other ideas include adding 1 tsp. mustard; making a thinner sauce by omitting the breadcrumbs; and adding some tiny pickled onions or 1 or 2 finely chopped gherkins to the blended sauce.*

Process 10 cups fresh flat-leaved parsley, 3/4 cup fresh basil leaves (optional), 5/8 cup canned anchovies, 3 Tbs. capers, 2 crushed garlic cloves, 1 Tbs. finely chopped shallots or onions, 4 Tbs. white breadcrumbs, and 3–4 Tbs. white wine vinegar in a blender or food processor. Trickle 1/2 cup olive oil into the mixture, and stir to make a smooth sauce—if it is too thick, dilute with a little more oil. Serve with raw or cooked vegetables, pasta or baked potatoes, or spread over whole-wheat bread or toast.

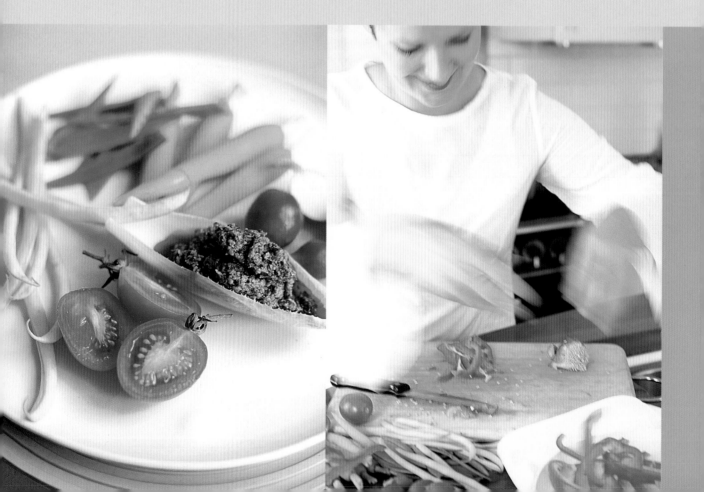

## SALSA ROSSA (SERVES 4)

In a saucepan, fry 1 minced onion and 1 chopped red pepper in 2 Tbs. olive oil until the onion and pepper are very soft, but not colored. Add 4 skinned, chopped tomatoes, sea salt, and hot chili powder to taste (the sauce should be quite peppery). Simmer for 30 minutes or until the liquid has reduced to a thick sauce.

## QUICK AND EASY MANGO SALSA (SERVES 4)

*Mangoes are full of cold-fighting vitamin C and take only a few minutes to process into a salsa. I think this tastes great with roast chicken, fish, or game.*

Peel and stone 1 large, ripe mango and then chop into small pieces. Transfer to a small bowl, and add 2 tsp. chopped fresh mint, 1 Tbs. lime juice, and 1 finely chopped small, red onion. Season to taste with a little sea salt, and some freshly ground black pepper. Refrigerate for 1 hour before serving.

## *herbal first aid for fevers*

Mix 10 drops of either wormwood or gentian tincture with water and take 3 times a day. Alternatively, make an infusion by adding 1 tsp. each yarrow and boneset to 1 cup of water with a pinch of cayenne pepper, then leave to infuse for 5 minutes before drinking. You can take up to 4 cups a day.

## BLACKBERRY AND PEACH DESSERT (SERVES 4)

**6 ripe peaches, skinned and stoned**　　**4 cups blackberries, washed**
**juice of 1 orange**　　**2 cups organic, live, natural yogurt**
**4 drops orange-blossom water**

Roughly slice the peaches and transfer to a blender. Add the orange juice and orange-blossom water, and blend until smooth. Spread a layer of blackberries over the bottom of four wineglasses or small glass dessert bowls. Spoon a layer of yogurt over the blackberries, followed by a layer of the peach blend. Continue layering in this way until you have used up all of the ingredients, reserving a couple of blackberries to pop on top of each dessert. Serve immediately.

## *herbal first aid for asthma, breathlessness and wheeziness*

Make an infusion using 1 handful each of nettle and thyme to 3 cups water to drink throughout the day. Another good remedy is German camomile: make an infusion by placing 2 heaped tsp. to 1 cup of water in a saucepan, covering and heating, then leaving it to stand for 10 minutes. Inhale the steam, then strain to make a fragrant, soothing tea. You could also use a couple of drops of camomile essential oil in a steam inhalation or on a clean cotton handkerchief.

# improving skin complaints and delaying aging

How your skin looks, in my opinion, gives a true indication of how healthy you are inside. Although living and working in today's polluted environments certainly hammer our complexions, whether you're worried about pimples, dry patches, or crow's feet around your eyes, your lifestyle and how you treat your body can have a huge impact on your skin's appearance, dramatically more so than expensive skin creams. Cherish your skin from the inside, and you'll save a fortune on potions and cosmetics.

This holistic approach is particularly important if you're anxious to fend off the signs of aging. In fact, the aging process receives an unfairly bad press when it comes to such skin changes as thinning and loss of elasticity, as well as the appearance of lines and wrinkles, which, in fact, have very little—if anything—do to with it. Although these changes typically become more obvious as we get older, aging isn't actually their cause. Think about it: while many eighty-year-olds have very smooth skin on some areas of their bodies, it's the parts that have been exposed to the sun over the course of a lifetime that are wrinkled, which just goes to show how severely the sun can damage the complexion. So protect your skin from the sun's harmful ultraviolet rays with sunscreen, and never bask in the sunshine between 11 A.M. and 3 P.M., when the sun is at its hottest. Defend your skin from the damaging free radicals that populate polluted environments, too, by supplying your body with plenty of skin-nurturing nutrients.

## 10 ways to flawless skin

Many skin complaints are caused, or exacerbated, by a lack or excess of certain nutrients, as well as certain lifestyle habits. I've identified ten key areas to tackle if you have troublesome skin.

1 Vitamin A can have a magical effect on problem skin, but don't apply any preparations containing it unless they've been prescribed by your doctor. Instead, boost your intake of foods that are rich in beta carotene (which the body converts into vitamin A), including carrots, watercress, apricots, mangoes, and melons.

2 Apricots, mangoes, and melons also contain high levels of vitamin C, one of the most effective skin-healers, as do blueberries, black currants, and blackberries (which also contain flavonoids), plums, papayas, and kiwi fruits, so tuck into these if your skin's playing up. If you smoke, you'll need to take a 2,000mg vitamin C supplement a day. Better still, do your skin an enormous favor and quit! Nicotine attacks the blood vessels that supply the skin with oxygen and nutrients, as well as those that drain away waste products, a buildup of which can aggravate pimples, eczema, and acne. What's more, smoking makes the skin leathery, somewhat like the effect that the curing, or smoking, process has on some fish.

3 Zinc reduces inflammatory processes within the body, so if your body is blighted by acne, eczema, or psoriasis, eat more zinc-rich foods, such as seafood, hard, crumbly cheeses, nuts, seeds, and legumes.

4 If you suffer from pimples, eczema, or psoriasis, also boost your intake of two further powerful anti-inflammatories—omega-3 fatty acid and eicosapentanoic acid—by eating oily fish (salmon, fresh tuna, sardines, or mackerel) twice a week. Omega-6 fatty acid can control the hormones that make the skin overly oily and consequently pimply. Put it to work for you by nibbling on foods that offer it, notably seeds such as linseeds, sunflower, sesame, pumpkin, and hemp, and nuts, which are also delicious roasted and sprinkled over cereals or salads.

5 Selenium and vitamin E are both skin-nurturing nutrients, so focus on eating the foods that contain them, including avocados, blackberries, mangoes, tomatoes, seeds, spinach, watercress, brazil nuts (a fantastic source of selenium), cashews, and wholewheat cereals.

6 Although it's a myth that sweet foods, such as chocolate, cause pimples, if they form a disproportionately large part of your diet, you probably aren't eating enough fruits and vegetables, a deficiency of which can cause problem skin; so if you're guilty of this, restore the balance.

7 The caffeine and tannins in tea, coffee, and colas dehydrate the skin, so don't drink more than a couple of these drinks a day. If you instead start drinking a daily 5 pints of water, your skin will reward you with a significant improvement in its appearance within only a few days.

8 Cut down your alcohol intake, because an overindulgence in booze, another dehydrator, can coarsen your skin and give you thread veins and open pores.

9 A poor complexion can sometimes be a sign that your gut isn't happy, particularly if you suffer from irritable-bowel syndrome (IBS). If you think that this may be the cause of your skin's distress, keep a note of everything that you eat and drink, as well as your skin's appearance, for a few weeks, to see if you can identify the food that may be irritating your digestive system and skin. Taking a probiotic, acidophilus supplement may also alleviate both problems.

10 Take regular cardiovascular exercise like running, cycling, or swimming (remember to wash your skin with pure water after getting out of the pool to flush away the chlorine and other chemical residues), which will pump a healthy supply of impurity-banishing blood around your skin. Try to get into a good, skin-nurturing sleeping routine, too (see pages 84–5).

# bodyfoods solutions for sparkling skin

### PAN-FRIED SALMON WITH LEMONY CHILI PASTA (SERVES 2)

*When cooking fish, I like to keep it simple. Here I have just pan-fried the salmon and served it with a basic fresh-tasting pasta. If you do not have preserved lemons, then use the zest and half the juice from 1 lemon.*

Bring a large pan of salted water to the boil, and drop in 7 oz. tagliatelle. Cook according to the instructions on the package. Meanwhile, heat a large skillet. Brush a little olive oil and seasoning over two salmon fillets and lay them in the pan. Fry for 3–4 minutes on each side until lightly golden or done to your liking. Remove from the pan and set aside to rest. Return the pan to the heat and add 2 Tbs. chopped capers, 3 Tbs. chopped preserved lemon, 1/2 tsp. crushed chili flakes and 2 Tbs. olive oil. Heat very gently for 2–3 minutes, then toss in the drained pasta. Spoon the tagliatelle into warmed pasta bowls, flake the salmon over, then sprinkle over 1 Tbs. roughly chopped parsley and a good grinding of black pepper. Serve immediately with a fresh green salad.

### ZESTY STEWED RHUBARB AND BLUEBERRIES (SERVES 4)

*Vitamin C is a key ingredient for nourishing your skin, and here's an easy way to combine fruits rich in this strong antioxidant. Rhubarb, orange, and blueberries make a lovely sharp, sweet, and tangy combination, which, in turn, is perfectly complemented by the whipped cream, ice milk, or fromage frais.*

Trim and wash 2 lb. rhubarb, then chop into bite-sized pieces and transfer to a pan. Sprinkle 1/8 cup fine granulated sugar, the zest and juice of 1 orange, and 1 tsp. ground ginger. Cover the pan and leave to cook over a gentle heat for 10–15 minutes or until the rhubarb has just softened, but still retains its shape. Remove the pan from the heat, and carefully stir in 1 cup fresh blueberries. Leave the fruit mixture to stand for about 15 minutes, or until the blueberries have softened and the mixture has cooled slightly. Serve warm or cold, layered in individual glasses with whipped cream, ice milk, or fromage frais, and perhaps with some brandy snaps or *langue de chat* cookies.

## MANGO, LIME, AND RASPBERRY JUICE (SERVES 2)

*Easy to make, this is great food for your skin, packed with masses of vitamin C and beta carotene.*

Peel ½ large, ripe mango and cut the flesh from the stone. Place in a blender with 20 large frozen raspberries, the juice of a large lime, and a few ice cubes if you like it chilled (otherwise add enough water to thin the mixture). Process together and serve.

## STRAWBERRIES WITH LEMON AND SUGAR (SERVES 4)

*Strawberries and cream is, of course, a classic combination and one of the quickest desserts to make; or you could team strawberries with black pepper, which really intensifies their flavor. If you prefer, you could steep them in orange juice or red wine.*

You'll need 1 1/2 lb. strawberries. Leave any small ones whole, and cut the larger ones into halves or quarters. Place in a bowl with the juice of 2 lemons and 3 Tbs. fine granulated sugar (or your preferred quantity). Stir them carefully, but thoroughly, to coat them with the sugar syrup, and leave them to sit for 20 minutes. Transfer to serving bowls and, if you like, serve with thick, Greek-style natural yogurt.

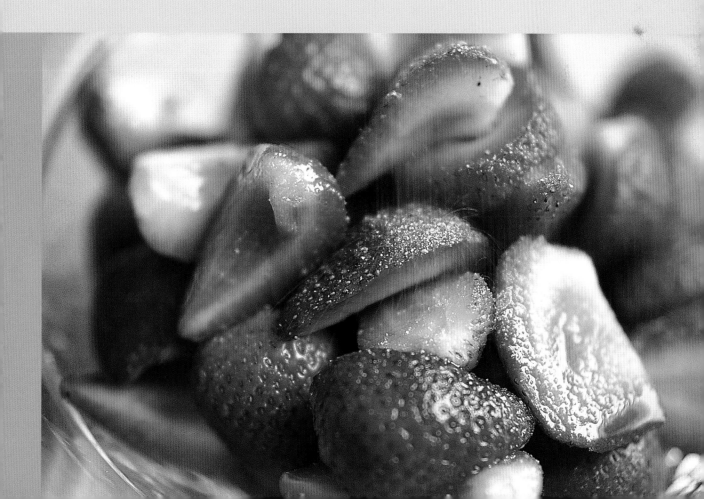

# dealing with IBS and digestive disorders

Developing irritable-bowel syndrome (IBS) is a very common way for a stressed body to react to a busy life. Even if you seem to be coping on the surface, you may still be bottling up your angst and exhaustion within your gut, which may respond by inflicting pain, bloating, diarrhea, constipation, nausea, and gas on you. An astounding 20 percent of the U.S. population is now said to suffer from IBS, a figure that I suspect will increase as our lives become ever more demanding.

On first receiving a diagnosis of IBS, many of my patients report having been told to eat more fiber and to learn to live with their distressing symptoms. In other cases, some doctors dash off a prescription without first having explored the individual's diet and lifestyle. Yet many people with IBS can alleviate their condition without recourse to drugs, simply by adjusting their eating habits and avoiding obviously stressful situations.

## eliminate common causes

One of the most common causes of IBS is intolerance of specific foods, notably wheat and dairy products. Cutting these two large food groups out of your diet can be problematic, so I'd first advise reducing your consumption, but then avoiding them altogether when you're feeling especially tired or stressed. Unless labeled wheat- or gluten-free, bread, cereals, pastries, pasta, sauces made with flour, and manufactured foods like sausages contain wheat. Gluten, a protein, is found in all grains, including wheat, barley, and rye, so that although all gluten-free foods are also wheat-free, not all wheat-free foods are gluten-free, because they may contain other grains. Gluten shouldn't cause you problems if you have IBS, but wheat may, so experiment to see whether reducing the amount of wheat in your diet helps (try having a couple of slices of toast for breakfast, for instance, and then avoiding wheat-containing foods for the rest of the day). Do the same with dairy products like milk, yogurt, butter, cream, and cheese, and remember that keeping a food-and-symptom diary for a few weeks is one of the best ways of monitoring your gut's reaction to a suspected trigger food.

IBS is sometimes aggravated by particularly fatty and rich foods like fried or creamy dishes, particularly if they also contain potatoes, cheese, onions, corn, or beef, or are enjoyed with white wine, all of which worsen IBS, as can drinking caffeine-rich coffee, tea, and cola. Having a cup of coffee can provoke a constipated gut to get moving in the morning, but don't risk it if your symptoms are making your life a misery. Instead, enlist the aid of mint and warmth, whether it be sipping a cup of warm mint tea, soaking in a warm bath or curling up with a hot-water bottle. If you don't like the taste of mint, try ginger, lemon verbena, or vervain (see page 13), all of which will soothe an irritated gut, unlike caffeine, which has the

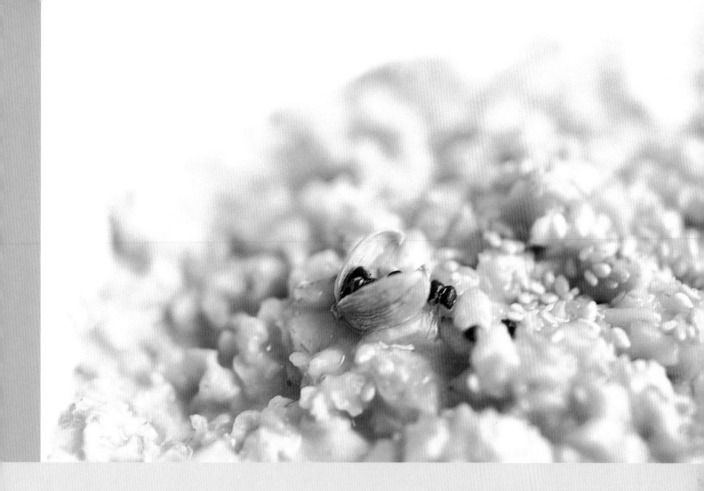

opposite effect. And if you stash a supply of herbal tea bags in your desk at work for emergency situations, you won't be tempted to subject your gut to caffeine when it's already under stress.

You may be able to tolerate fruits and vegetables—particularly if they're cooked—white bread, pasta or rice, so experiment to see which suits you best, but steer clear of carbonated drinks and lots of high-fiber, whole-grain or raw foods, which can be too challenging for an IBS-stricken gut to cope with. Bran-based cereals are incredibly hard for IBS sufferers to digest, and may even cause serious complications, so give bran a wide berth and instead opt for a gentler, wholewheat cereal, a granola containing such seeds, as linseeds or pumpkin seeds, or my fragrant Cardamom Rice Milk Porridge (see page 42).

On a more positive note, drinking at least 5 pints water a day will also alleviate your symptoms. It doesn't matter if the water is hot or cold, although some IBS sufferers find that they tolerate room-temperature water better than ice-cold or piping-hot water.

## *herbal first aid for digestive disorders*

Drinking anise, cardamom, fennel, lemon verbena, or peppermint tea may help to alleviate gas and bloating.

# calming heartburn and indigestion

Following the guidelines given for IBS on pages 98–9 will also help to avert both heartburn and indigestion, but sometimes there's no escaping them. When either strikes, avoid acidic foods like vinegar and pickles and such overly fatty foods as French fries, potato chips, nuts, and rich, creamy, or fried foods. Some of my patients also find that raw vegetables, particularly chilies, peppers, onions, and garlic, and citrus or unripe fruits sit heavily in the stomach, causing acid reflux.

If you're prone to indigestion, above all, try to eat slowly and in as relaxed an environment as possible. As madly busy as life can be, if you remove yourself from the hustle and bustle for 5–10 minutes, banish your worries from your mind, and really concentrate on enjoying your food, eating it slowly, chewing it thoroughly, and savoring every mouthful, your gut will stick to digesting, not "indigesting." Sipping fennel, mint, apple, or camomile tea also helps to keep your stomach on your side. And, however late you return home, taking a few minutes at the end of a hectic working day to relax before eating, perhaps by having a bath or shower, will prepare your stomach to digest your supper much better than hurtling to the fridge as soon as you walk through the door. Other tips include not drinking too much (of anything) while you're eating and stopping smoking.

Finally, some instances of indigestion are related to the presence of *Helicobacter pylori* bacteria in the digestive system, so if your indigestion persists, ask your doctor for a breath test. If the test confirms the diagnosis, you may be prescribed antibiotics. Alternatively, having 1 tsp. Manuka honey, containing live UMF factor, twice a day (either as it is or mixed with yogurt, but don't heat it), or a daily dose of 1g mastic gum, for two weeks can help to eradicate the bacteria.

## *herbal first aid for digestive disorders*

Constipation: dandelion root, licorice, and yellow dock are mild laxatives, while senna is more powerful and should be taken only when other herbs have failed to work. (Caution: don't take senna, yellow dock, or licorice if you're pregnant.)

Cramp: bark has antispasmodic properties and can soothe colicky, spasm-type constipation.

Psyllium husks and seeds encourage normal bowel habits by cleansing the colon.

Agrimony, sage, bistort, and black catechu all target diarrhea. You can make a decoction by adding 1 heaped tsp. of any of these herbs to 1 1/2 cups of water in a saucepan, and letting this simmer over a low heat for 15–20 minutes. Take up to 3 cups a day for no longer than three days. (Caution: don't take sage if you're pregnant.)

## CHICKEN WITH WINTER VEGETABLES (SERVES 4)

*Sometimes our bodies just want simple, easy-to-digest meals, and they couldn't come better than this.*

1 medium-sized organic chicken

1 large bunch flat-leaved parsley

4 bunches thyme

3 bay leaves

small head of fennel, finely minced

3 leeks, cleaned and roughly chopped

4 carrots, peeled and roughly chopped

small head of celery root, roughly chopped

1 bottle dry white wine

sea salt and freshly ground black pepper

1 lb. small, waxy potatoes, peeled

Heat the oven to 400°. Remove the giblets and wash the chicken well. Place in a large, earthenware casserole with a lid. Separate the parsley leaves from their stalks and set both aside. Throw the thyme, bay leaves, parsley stalks, and vegetables into the casserole. Pour in the wine and season with a little sea salt and plenty of black pepper. Cover and cook, in the middle of the oven, for 2½ hours. When the chicken is cooked, remove and discard the parsley stalks. Transfer the chicken to a serving plate and cover with plastic wrap. Now boil the potatoes until cooked. Finely chop the reserved parsley leaves and add to the cooked vegetables, check the seasoning, and stir well. The best way of serving this dish is to savor the thick parsley-and-vegetable soup to start with and then to move on to the room-temperature chicken, accompanied by the potatoes, with a little light Dijon mustard on the side.

## KEDGEREE (SERVES 4–6)

2 lb. finnan haddie or smoked salmon

2 bay leaves

5/8 cup basmati rice

3/4 stick unsalted butter

6 green onions, minced

1 small garlic clove, minced

2 tsp. medium-strength curry powder

juice of 2 lemons

3 Tbs. chopped cilantro

3 organic eggs, hard boiled

Place the fish in a large, deep skillet. Add the bay leaves and a little water, to half the depth of the pan. Bring to the boil, then turn down and simmer for about 5 minutes or until the fish is poached (it should turn cloudy). Transfer the fish to a small bowl, remove the skin and flake into chunks. In a separate pan, boil the rice for about 10 minutes until cooked, then drain well. Clean and dry the skillet, put it back on the heat, and add the butter. Gently sauté the onions and garlic until clear and soft. Add the curry powder and cook for 2 minutes. Add the fish, rice, and half the lemon juice, mixing gently, but thoroughly. Stirring constantly, ensure all the ingredients are hot, then remove from the heat and add the cilantro. Season to taste, then transfer to a warmed serving dish. Slice the boiled eggs into quarters and arrange on top. Sprinkle the remaining lemon juice over and serve at once.

# coping with premenstrual syndrome

A staggering 40–90 percent of women experience PMS on a regular basis, with the largest number being in their thirties and forties. For years, women were told it was "all in their heads"; but thank goodness, research now backs us, showing that there is a physiological cause.

It's normally due to a combination of hormonal imbalances, fluid and salt retention, alterations in chemicals such as prostaglandins, which affect our nervous system, low blood sugar, and, last but by no means least, nutrient shortages or excesses. The food and drink you consume before and especially during this time can have a massive effect on whether or not you become—or feel—like a monster! If premenstrual syndrome (PMS) blights your every month, following these tips may help you to weather the worst of the hormonal storm.

## survival tips for that time of the month

- Boost your intake of inflammation-soothing omega oils by eating oily fish, such as fresh tuna, salmon, herrings, mackerel, and sardines, as often as you can, and incorporating seeds and nuts into your diet.
- Eat little and often. The best snacks to nibble on between meals include fresh fruits, nuts, roasted seeds, and small tubs of live yogurt.
- Avoid very salty foods, which aggravate fluid retention, and also overly sweet foods. If the urge to comfort yourself with a dose of chocolate is overwhelming, carrying a small bottle of vanilla essence around with you and having a sniff whenever the craving hits really helps to satisfy your chocolate lust, without saddling your body with excess calories.
- Reduce your consumption of alcohol and caffeine-containing drinks—better still, cut them out altogether—which only make you feel ten times more hormonal and ratty.
- Visit your health-food store for supplements that target PMS, notably those based on evening primrose oil or linseed oil.
- For me, swimming is one of the best strategies to help me survive the mood swings. There is something very comforting and cocooning about feeling the water wash over your body.
- Mark your PMS days in your diary so that you can keep high-stress activities well away from them. Have a massage—or just take time for yourself, so that you're not fighting your PMS symptoms. Try to switch off, concentrate on your breathing, meditate—the calmer you can stay, the less you will suffer.

## herbal first aid for PMS

Make an infusion of either vervain or lime, or an equal mixture of both (you can drink up to 5 cups a day). If your menstrual cycle is irregular, take 1.5–2ml *Agnus castus* tincture with water each morning on waking—for at least two months—to help your body to settle into a more regular rhythm. For external application, add 5–10 drops of rosemary essential oil to your bathwater.

## 5 ways to reduce fluid retention

If you suffer from swollen and sore breasts, a common condition caused by fluid retention, following these nutritional strategies may ease your discomfort.

1 As illogical as it may sound, drink plenty of water or herbal teas (see pages 12–13). The herbs dandelion, nettle, fennel, and parsley are especially effective when it comes to encouraging your body to relinquish excess fluid.

2 Focus on eating citrus fruits and melon, asparagus, watercress, cucumber, and fennel. Alternatively, try liquidizing these fresh vegetables to make healthy, breast-soothing juices. All of this fresh produce contains vitamin C and plenty of water, which help the body to produce anti-inflammatory substances and relieve fluid retention.

3 Up your intake of potassium-packed foods like bananas, tomatoes, and whole grains.

4 Include lots of vitamin E-rich foods in your diet, such as seeds, nuts, brown rice, asparagus, avocados, salmon, and sardines.

5 Boost your magnesium intake by incorporating bulgur wheat, lentils, and other legumes into your meals.

# improving fertility and conception

The areas that stressful, busy lives seem to hit particularly hard are sexuality and fertility: the harder and longer hours we work, the less we take care of our bodies and the more difficulty we have conceiving. Sexuality is a complex and sensitive issue, and a loss of libido can have many causes. Because partnership difficulties often manifest themselves in bed, psychosexual problems may be a significant factor, but if a relationship is healthy, the problem may be rooted in the body rather than the mind, which is where nutrients can come to the rescue.

Researchers still can't explain why, but I'm nevertheless convinced that if couples don't take enough time to eat, drink, and rest properly, loading themselves with modern-day body drainers like being overweight, drinking too much alcohol and coffee, and smoking, their bodies will become drained of essential fertility-boosting nutrients—although none of these factors can be exclusively blamed for infertility.

## get in the mood

When couples come to see me with fertility difficulties, the first thing I ask is how much sex they're having. As obvious as it may sound, this issue is often passed over, yet our sex lives can be eroded by a number of factors. Research has shown that the rate of conception is lowered if either partner—or both—is carrying weight in excess of the ideal body-mass-index (BMI) range of 25–25 (or, alternatively, if the figure stands below 20). Fertility is, of course, inextricably linked with libido, and a woman who is overweight may feel undesirable and consequently not in the mood for sex, while an obese man's weight may hamper his performance. So if weight is contributing to a reduced libido or an inability to conceive, losing it gradually—about a 2 lb. a week—by having a well-balanced diet and exercising regularly may do the trick. Swimming is one of the best libido-enhancing exercises of all because the cool water encourages your body to produce the sex-boosting hormone norepinephrine, as do arguing, mild pain—and exposure to danger! (See also pages 116–19 for some weight-loss recipes and ideas.)

Leading stressful lives can also eat away at sexual desire. When you're feeling constantly tired and drained, your energy levels may be so low that by the time you reach the bedroom all you want to do is go to sleep. How dark or light your bedroom is can have an impact on your libido, too, because dim winter days and dark winter nights (and bedrooms) stimulate your body to generate melatonin, a hormone that makes you want to sleep. This soporific state can be reinforced by eating too many starchy, high-carbohydrate foods, so that after sharing a big bowl of pasta on a winter's evening all that you'll be up to is a quick cuddle before going to sleep. Conversely, light can bring melatonin production to a halt, causing your libido to shoot upward. If it's stimulation and stamina that you require from your food, opt for a meal that includes a concentrated source of protein, such as chicken served with roasted vegetables, or an omelet or steak with salad. Remember, too, that overeating and drinking too much alcohol will both make you want to conk out. Ginger tea (simply made from grating fresh gingerroot in boiling water) helps digestion and can also energize you.

## go nuts

Over the past few years, one nutrient has shot to the forefront of fertility research, namely selenium, a mineral that is essential for fertility. Indeed, in a recent study of Scottish men, selenium supplements were shown to increase their sperm motility significantly, indicating that they had been selenium deficient.

We don't yet know enough about how much selenium we should have in our diet—although we think it's in the region of 60–70mg a day—to recommend supplements, so, instead, I'd advocate boosting your intake of the most concentrated dietary sources of selenium. These include brazil nuts (which offer 1,530mg per 100g), mixed nuts and raisins (170mg), dried mushrooms (110mg), lentils (105mg), and canned tuna (80mg). In practice, this could mean having brazil nuts and raisins as a snack, chopping them and sprinkling them over your cereal, making granola (see page 42), or using canned (dolphin-friendly) tuna in sandwiches, as well as varying your diet to include other selenium-providers, such as squid (delectable in risotto nero), flounder, sole, sardines, and swordfish. Too much selenium is toxic; however, and the current recommendation is to take no more than 440mg a day, which equates to roughly 1/4 cup brazil nuts or 1 3/4 cups mixed nuts and raisins.

Zinc, vitamin C, and vitamin E are also linked with infertility and libido, which makes it vital to have a generally well-balanced diet that is rich in fresh fruits, vegetables, whole grains, nuts, seeds, and legumes, because this will give you all three. A zinc deficiency has been shown to cause low sperm counts and motility; vitamin C has been found to increase sperm production and decrease sperm stickiness, thereby improving the chances of conception; while vitamin E is vital for the development and maintenance of strong cells, particularly in the blood, and for helping the sperm to penetrate the egg.

Women who are hoping to become mothers may be interested to learn that the herb *Agnus castus* has been shown to enhance fertility, possibly through its ability to normalize levels of the hormone progesterone—required for the maintenance of pregnancy—within the body. And external use of rose oil is thought to help ensure regular menstrual cycles. Overheated testes have been shown to reduce sperm production, so men should keep their testes cool by avoiding tight-fitting trousers and taking showers, rather than baths. Also for men, hemp oil is rich in essential omega oils, which help produce prostaglandins—present in semen—and also to manufacture sex hormones. It has a strong taste, and can't be heated, so try using it half and half with a light olive oil in salad dressings.

# bodyfoods solutions for boosting fertility

## CHICKEN WITH CHICKPEAS AND BAY (SERVES 4)

2 Tbs. olive oil

3 small shallots, finely minced

1 small leek, minced

1 medium-sized carrot, minced

2 stalks celery, minced

2 large garlic cloves, minced

a handful of chopped cilantro

3¼-lb. free-range, organic chicken, washed
   and cut into 8 pieces

4 bay leaves

sea salt and freshly ground black pepper

1¼ cups chickpeas, drained and washed

generous ⅝ cup dry white wine

Gently heat the oil in a skillet large enough to hold the chicken pieces in a single layer, without overlapping. Add the shallots and cook over a medium heat until golden brown. Add the leek, carrot, celery, and garlic, and cook for another 5 minutes, stirring frequently to prevent sticking. Add the cilantro and the chicken pieces, skin down. Cook the chicken until brown on the skin side, turn over, and cook until the other side browns, too. Add the bay leaves, some sea salt and plenty of freshly ground black pepper, stirring well to ensure that all the chicken pieces are coated. Cook for another 10 minutes, then add the chickpeas and the wine. Continue cooking for another 5 minutes, stirring well to combine the caramelized vegetables, chicken juices, and wine. Once you've smelled the alcohol evaporate, which will take just a few minutes, turn down the heat and cover the pan with a lid. Cook for another 40 minutes, stirring occasionally to prevent sticking, until the chicken is thoroughly cooked (no longer pink) and easily falls away from the bone. Remove and discard the bay leaves. Check the seasoning before serving.

## OYSTERS (SERVES 2)

*We don't still believe in the concept of aphrodisiac foods, but coincidentally not only are oysters very sexy to eat but they're also oozing with zinc, a mineral that can have a positive effect on both conception and fertility. To be as sure as possible that they are fresh, always buy oysters from a reliable source, and look for a tightly closed shell, a sign of freshness. You can store tightly closed oysters in a deep bowl covered, with a wet, clean dish towel, in the fridge for a few hours, until you're ready to scrub and eat them.*

Opening oysters can be a little tricky. The best and safest way is to hold the oyster, with the unhinged part of the shell pointing downward, in a clean cloth in the palm of your hand. Using an oyster knife, pry open the shell at its hinge, working the knife point into it until you've cut the ligament. (I prefer to remove

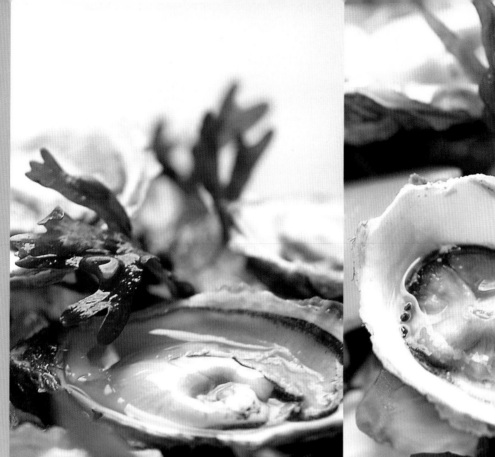
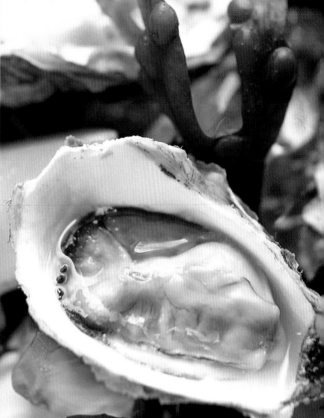

the beard, but you don't have to.) Now loosen the oyster, but leave it in the shell, swimming in its own juices. Serve the oyster cold (on crushed ice if possible), but eat it whichever way you like!

## VANILLA ROSE FRUIT SALAD (SERVES 4)

*We all know fresh fruits are good for us, but they can sometimes be a little too predictable. Here's a quick and easy way to jazz them up and enjoy a dessert without feeling guilty. You can choose from a large variety of fruits; I use about 1 lb. 10 oz. of a mixture of nectarines, strawberries, raspberries, peaches, and cherries. This recipe will serve four, but you could instead make it just for yourself and keep it in the fridge for a couple of days, so that you can repeatedly go back for more!*

Place 2 Tbs. redcurrant jelly, 1 Tbs. clear honey, 1 split vanilla pod and 3/4 cup water (or, if you prefer, dessert wine) in a small pan, and bring the mixture to the boil. Remove the pan from the heat and leave the mixture to infuse for 15 minutes. Then remove the vanilla pod and stir in 1 Tbs. rosewater. Meanwhile, wash your chosen fruits and cut them into bite-sized pieces. Transfer the fruit to a serving bowl, pour the warm fragrant liquid over, and leave the fruit salad to cool and the flavors to blend for a while. Then refrigerate it until you're ready to enjoy it or in need of a fruit boost.

# nurturing your body
# through pregnancy

If you're planning to conceive in the near future, now's a good time to take stock of your health and lifestyle and to focus on getting your body into a fit, well-nourished condition. Many women find that if this time is spent looking after themselves and feeling good, the period prior to pregnancy is very empowering.

Along with eating well and exercising, the main areas to target include giving up smoking and, if necessary, either shedding or gaining a few extra pounds, because having a body-mass index (BMI) of over 25 or under 20 reduces your chance of conception. Not only will these measures benefit your health, when you do conceive, they'll cut the risk of your baby being born underweight or with birth defects. The issue of alcohol is controversial. Although some authorities regard 7 drinks per week as a safe upper limit, I'd advise avoiding it altogether—apart, perhaps, from the occasional celebratory drink.

Having a well-balanced diet is important, as is ensuring that it includes plenty of foods that are rich in folic acid. Low folate levels have been linked with babies being born with such neural-tube defects as spina bifida. You should therefore be eating lots of fruits, nuts, green vegetables such as asparagus, fresh orange juice, fortified breakfast cereals, and beans for at least three months before conceiving, and should also take a daily supplement of 400mg of folic acid. Occasionally folic acid may cause sickness and diarrhea—if so, try splitting your dose in half and spacing out when you take it, or discuss different brands with your pharmacist. Rarely, you may have to rely just on diet to boost folic acid levels, but talk to your doctor if folic acid doesn't suit you. Laying down additional stores of calcium and iron—minerals that your body draws upon heavily during pregnancy—by eating the appropriate foods (see pages 36–9) will also stand you in good stead.

## when you're pregnant

Mothers-to-be usually ask me how much they should be eating in order to provide their unborn babies with the nutrients they need. The body generally doesn't require increased supplies of nutrients because it adapts to pregnancy by becoming more efficient at absorbing them from the gut. If you start eating for two, you'll spend months trying to regain your figure after your baby's birth. It may surprise you to learn that the body requires only an additional 200 calories per day during the last three months of pregnancy (equating to $7/8$ cup milk or a couple of large bananas).

There are, however, three nutrients that your body requires more of during pregnancy: calcium (which, from the time of conception until you stop breast-feeding, is leached out of your bones to provide for your growing baby), vitamin C, and vitamin D, all of which you'll receive if you boost your intake of dairy products, fresh fruits, vegetables, and oily fish, such as salmon, fresh tuna, sardines, and mackerel. On the subject of oily fish, research has linked a diet that is rich in the essential fatty acids (EFAs) that they contain with a reduced risk of developing high blood pressure, a longer pregnancy, and consequently a baby with a high birth weight and optimal brain and eye development. It's therefore vital to eat lots of EFAs (which seeds and nuts, and their oils, such as hemp or linseed, also contain) during the last trimester, when your unborn baby's brain increases dramatically in size. Conversely, make a concerted effort to avoid foods that are rich in trans-fatty acids (labeled in processed foods as vegetable fat or partially hydrogenated vegetable oil), an overconsumption of which has been linked with premature death, low birth weight, and a high risk of brain damage among newborns. Keep to frequent small meals to avoid indigestion and hunger pangs—both can cripple a pregnant stomach (see page 59 for healthy snacks).

## food safety

Food safety, a key concern for mothers-to-be, is relatively straightforward. Simply avoid the following:

- Raw or lightly cooked eggs and anything containing them, such as mayonnaise, mousses, and tiramisu, because they pose a salmonella risk.
- Pâté and all products that contain liver, to avoid overdosing on vitamin A and to fend off listeria.
- Soft, mold-ripened cheeses, both pasteurized and unpasteurized, such as blue cheeses and soft goat cheeses, to avert the danger of contracting listeria. (Hard cheeses—even unpasteurized ones like Parmesan—are fine.)
- Raw and partly cooked meat, fish, and poultry (including sushi, sashimi, steak tartare, oysters, and other types of raw seafood), as well as unpasteurized milk, to ward off toxoplasmosis and other bacterial infections.
- Prepackaged or deli salads and dressings, to protect yourself from listeria. (Pre-prepared salad leaves sold in bags can be safe, however, as long as you rinse them thoroughly under cold running water.)
- Excessive amounts of caffeine-containing drinks, like coffee and tea, to avoid upsetting your energy levels and moods. More importantly, drinking more than 5 cups a day increases the risk of miscarriage. It's therefore best to switch to herbal teas (see page 13), and if you're feeling nauseous, an infusion of grated gingerroot or freshly squeezed lemon juice may settle your stomach.

## weighting game

Another worrying issue for expectant mothers is weight gain. Although there are no absolutes, if your BMI was lower than 20 at conception, expect to put on 27½–40 lb.; if it was 20–26, 25–35 lb.; and if it was 26–30, 15–25 lb. If your BMI was over 30, you'll be expected to put on a minimum of 13 lb., with your obstetrician monitoring you carefully to ensure you don't gain too much weight, which increases the risk of complications caused by high blood pressure (preeclampsia) and pregnancy-onset diabetes. It's best to gain weight slowly, but steadily, during your pregnancy.

# bodyfoods solutions for mothers-to-be

### RED-BERRY SODA (SERVES 2)

*Although it's best to avoid alcohol when pregnant, it can be a real bore drinking yet more carbonated water. Here are two nonalcoholic drinks to liven up your evening that take only minutes to prepare.*

Purée 1¼ cups raspberries with 1 Tbs. lemon juice. Sieve 1 Tbs. confectioners' sugar into the purée, and stir gently. Put some ice cubes into the bottom of two glasses and divide the purée between each. Add ½ cup cranberry juice to each glass and top with soda water or carbonated water. Serve immediately.

### BLACKBERRY, RASPBERRY, AND MINT COCKTAIL (SERVES 2)

Place two large glass tumblers in the freezer. In a small bowl, combine two handfuls of blackberries, another two of raspberries, and the juice of a lemon. Using a fork, gently mush the fruits together until the mixture is almost smooth. Finely chop a sprig of mint and gently stir into the fruit. Transfer the fruit mixture to the frozen tumblers, add a few ice cubes, top with soda water or sparkling water and drink at once.

### CHICKPEA SOUP (SERVES 4)

*Some people think dried legumes are too much of a bother, but all that you have to do is soak them the night before you want to use them. The taste of home-cooked beans is wonderfully nutty and so superior that I think it's worth the little extra effort; this recipe is also very sustaining.*

**3/8 cup dried chickpeas, soaked overnight in cold water**

**4 garlic cloves**

**4 Tbs. olive oil**

**2 oz. pancetta, chopped into small pieces**

**2 tsp. fresh rosemary, minced**

**5/8 cup canned plum tomatoes, roughly chopped, with their juices**

**1¼ cup chicken, beef, or vegetable stock**

**sea salt and freshly ground black pepper**

Heat the oven to 325°. Drain the chickpeas and rinse them in fresh cold water, then place in a medium-sized casserole dish that is suitable for use both on the burner and in the oven. Add enough water to cover the chickpeas by 1 in. Place the casserole dish on the burner and bring the water to the boil. Cover the dish with a lid, and transfer it to the oven's middle shelf for 1½ hours or until the chickpeas are tender. Remove from the oven. In a medium-sized saucepan, sauté the garlic in the olive oil until dark golden brown. Remove and discard the garlic, leaving as much olive oil in the pan as possible. Add the pancetta to the pan and cook until golden brown. Now add the rosemary, tomatoes,

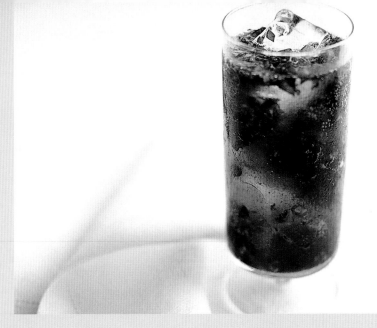

and their juices, and stir well. Cover and leave to simmer for 30 minutes, stirring occasionally. Drain the chickpeas, add to the pancetta mixture, stir, and cook for another 2 minutes. Pour in the stock and cook for a final 20 minutes. Season to taste with a little sea salt and plenty of freshly ground black pepper.

## CUCUMBER AND HERB SALAD (SERVES 6)

*A simple refreshing salad that can liven up pregnancy-dulled taste buds.*

Peel a cucumber and slice it finely. Arrange the cucumber slices on a large dinner or soup plate, and sprinkle evenly with 1 level tsp. fine sea salt. Place a large plate on top of the slices, and weight it down with a heavy can (this, along with the salt, will force the cucumber slices to relinquish their juices). After about 30 minutes, drain off the cucumber liquid, rinse the slices, and then pat them with paper towels until they are thoroughly dry. Transfer the cucumber slices, to a shallow dish. Sprinkle with 2 Tbs. tarragon vinegar, 1/2 tsp. fine granulated sugar and 2 level tsp. chopped fresh chives and mix well. Season to taste with freshly ground black pepper and fine granulated sugar before serving.

## *herbal first aid for morning sickness*

- For the first three months of pregnancy, take camomile tea (make an infusion in a covered container) in small quantities throughout the day, but don't drink more than 5 cups a day.
- Try making an infusion of 1/2 tsp. fennel seeds per cup of water (you can drink up to 3 cups a day).

## *herbal first aid for stretch marks*

- For external application only: rub aloe vera gel over the affected area.
- Try massaging olive oil all over your body up to twice a day to avert more stretch marks—a good excuse for much needed time to yourself.

# correcting hormonal and thyroid imbalances

"Your hormones must be playing up" are words that we never like to hear, because they make us feel disempowered. This needn't be the case, however, because whether your thyroid gland is misbehaving or your body is going through the menopause, how you eat and live your life can have a major impact on how you feel and, consequently, look.

The years between 55 and 60 are often among the most hormonally challenging for women, being the time when they usually enter the menopause—as, increasingly, do many men (although this is a controversial issue).

## the menopause and andropause

For women, the hormonal changes brought about by the menopause cause a gradual decline in fertility, spelling an end to their ability to bear children naturally, as well as hitting them with a host of unpleasant symptoms, ranging from the mildly disruptive to the life-wrecking. Such menopausal manifestations include hot flashes, extreme tiredness, dramatic mood swings, depression, libido problems, and insomnia. These may also affect men undergoing the male menopause, or andropause, who may additionally suffer increased hair loss and impotence.

Although hormone-replacement therapy (HRT)—estrogen therapy for women and testosterone therapy for men—can alleviate these symptoms, it is associated with some significant potential drawbacks, such as an increased risk of developing breast cancer and heart disease and of suffering strokes (although it is thought to reduce the incidence of bowel cancer, bone fractures, and Alzheimer's disease) among women, and a higher-than-average chance of developing prostate cancer and blood clots, in turn leading to strokes and heart attacks, among men.

The good news is that whether or not you decide to opt for HRT, taking certain dietary measures can have a positive impact on your symptoms, as well as fending off those "big" conditions to which you become increasingly vulnerable as you grow older—namely, arthritis and diabetes, osteoporosis (brittle-bone disease), heart disease, strokes (see pages 120–27), and cancer (see pages 128–31).

If you're a woman, boost your consumption of soy-based foods (like tofu and soy yogurt and milk). Soy, like other estrogenic foods, such as legumes, linseeds (delicious roasted), bean sprouts (add them to stir-fries and salads), and other fresh vegetables, contains potent phyto-estrogens, which can counteract the symptoms that are caused when your body's estrogen levels drop.

If you're a man, the advice is less clear-cut, but the healthier your diet, the less you'll suffer the symptoms of the andropause, so eat as much fresh produce as possible, quit smoking, and reduce your intake of saturated animal fats (including red meat, butter, cream, cheese, and fatty meats), alcohol and caffeine-containing drinks.

Whether you're male or female, giving up caffeine is one of the best things that you can do for your body, and not only in terms of weathering the menopause or andropause. Instead, switch to lattes made with decaffeinated coffee (the milk will provide calcium, a nutrient that plays a vital role in warding off osteoporosis) and fruit smoothies made with soy milk; and, of course, drink 5 pints of water each day. Get regular exercise, such as walking briskly, swimming, or cycling.

My parting tip is to eat lots of vitamin E-rich food such as olive oil, seeds, nuts, whole grains, cabbage, tuna preserved in oil, and asparagus, as well as oily fish like sardines, tuna, and mackerel, which contain omega-3 fatty acids. And if you're interested in exploring the herbal route, I'd recommend black cohosh, sage, *Agnus castus,* and red claw.

## hypothyroidism

The chief function of the thyroid gland, which is situated in the throat, just above the breastbone, is metabolic—it regulates body temperature, along with the rate at which the body burns heat- and energy-providing fuel, by secreting the hormone thyroxin. If it produces insufficient thyroxin (the condition known as hypothyroidism), the result can be a mishmash of distressing symptoms, including exhaustion, weight gain, hair loss, a diminished libido, depression, a high blood-cholesterol level, constipation, and bloating, swelling around the eyes and ankles and a husky, low voice. If these symptoms strike a chord with you, try a simple test that you can carry out at home by taking your temperature before getting out of bed in the morning. Leave the thermometer under your arm for 15 minutes. If the reading is then below 97.4°, it may be an indication that your thyroid gland is not functioning normally, in which case consult your doctor.

If you are diagnosed with hypothyroidism, your doctor may prescribe synthetic thyroxin. Alternatively, certain herbal and nutritional treatments may help you to manage your condition, the best known being to eat seaweed (also known as kelp or bladderwrack), which contains iodine, a nutrient that the thyroid gland needs in order to manufacture thyroxin. Bugleweed (wonderful name!) has sedative properties and is used for the opposite problem—an overactive thyroid gland, which has symptoms such as anxiety and weight loss (see pages 114–15 for nutrition ideas). Consult your doctor or medicinal herbalist before taking any herbal remedy, including an iodine supplement, to make sure that it suits your thyroid-gland status.

# bodyfoods solutions for hormone imbalances

### RAW VEGETABLES DIPPED IN OLIVE OIL (SERVES 4)

*Raw vegetables are low in calories, but high in vitamins and minerals.*

Quarter 2 fennel bulbs and break up 1 small celery head. Halve 2 large carrots and 2 very small cucumbers lengthwise. Arrange these raw vegetables on a plate with 8 green onions. In a small bowl, beat a little sea salt and freshly ground black pepper into $5/8$ cup extra-virgin olive oil, then transfer to a serving dish. Serve the raw vegetables with the olive-oil dip and fresh bread.

### CHICKEN AND BACON SALAD WITH HONEY MUSTARD DRESSING (SERVES 2)

**6 strips smoked bacon**

**1 bag mixed salad leaves**

**a handful of cherry tomatoes, halved**

**1 chicken breast, roasted, the skin removed
  and shredded**

**1 avocado, peeled, stoned, and sliced**

*For the dressing*

**2 Tbs. clear honey**

**4 Tbs. olive oil**

**1 Tbs. white wine vinegar**

**1 Tbs. grainy mustard**

**sea salt and freshly ground black pepper**

Lay the bacon in a skillet over a medium heat and cook until light golden and crisp. Remove from the pan and transfer to a few pieces of paper towel to absorb any excess fat. Tip the salad leaves into a shallow serving bowl. Add the cherry tomatoes, roast chicken breast, and avocado. To make the dressing, mix together the honey, olive oil, vinegar, mustard, and a little sea salt and plenty of freshly ground black pepper to taste. When you are ready to eat, pour the dressing over the salad leaves and toss them well. Break the crisp bacon into pieces and sprinkle them over the salad. Serve immediately, perhaps with some warmed ciabatta bread.

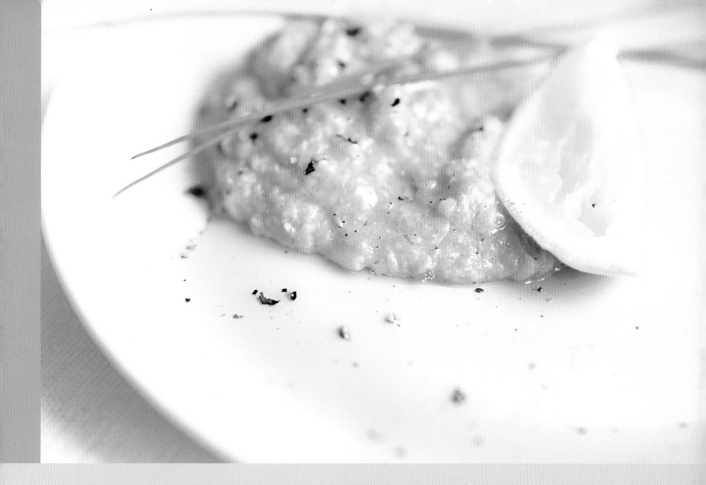

## FAVA BEAN PURÈE (SERVES 4)

*Cooking dried beans may appear too much effort, but it only takes the inclination to think a little way ahead. It's so worth the effort, as you'll be left with a dish that tastes delicious as well as being very healthful.*

The day before making this dish, soak 2 cups skinned, dried fava beans in cold water overnight. The next day, drain the beans and place them in a saucepan with 2 chopped celery stalks, 1 chopped large potato, and 2 chopped medium-sized onions. Cover the vegetables with water, bring the water to the boil, and then cook over a low heat for about 2 hours. Toward the end of the cooking time, add some sea salt and a little olive oil, stirring the mixture thoroughly. Transfer the mixture to a food processor and purée it. Now beat in $1/2$ cup olive oil. Serve immediately.

## GINGER, ORANGE, AND MINT SMOOTHIE (SERVES 1)

*This juice will help to lift you out of the hormonal doldrums and calm your digestion.*

Peel and grate a small knob of fresh ginger, saving the juice. Squeeze 4 medium-sized organic oranges, and pour the juice into a blender, along with the ginger pulp and juice. Add 8 large, washed mint leaves and blend thoroughly.

# boosting weight loss and avoiding weight gain

The first step on the path to losing weight is to recognize that what works for someone else may not suit you. Becoming stressed out about sticking to a punishing diet because some celebrity endorses it, is not going to get you anywhere, not least because feeling ravenous, light-headed, and grouchy seriously affects your ability to cope with the demands of a busy life. So ignore the lure of the quick-fix diet and, instead, accept that you'll need to embrace the weight-loss lifestyle.

I've noticed that stressed-out, busy people tend to turn to food and drink as their main sources of relaxation at the end of yet another frantic day. But if you're hoping to lose weight, try to build a more life-affirming activity into your evenings, such as meditating, reading for pleasure, or phoning friends; the more you can do to make your life well rounded, the less you'll want to seek solace in food. The best thing that you can do for both mind and body is to exercise (after all, losing weight is all about burning up more calories than you consume), so aim to get 20 minutes of steady exercise three times a week.

Rather than becoming fixated on achieving a particular weight, the crucial thing is to stay positive by envisioning your body looking slimmer and healthier. How you feel in yourself is far more important than how much you weigh, so maximize the feel-good factor by enhancing your assets (how about some sexy underwear?). Be realistic: your body is likely to be either an apple or a pear shape, and, although you can become a smaller apple or pear, you'll never be able to switch to the other camp. If you want to monitor your progress, ignore the scale and instead measure your waist, thighs, and arms with a tape measure, draw a picture of yourself, and then record your dimensions on it in inches. This way, you'll be focusing on your change in shape, which most of us care far more about than what the scales tell us.

A few other tips include juggling tastes and textures within a meal, to keep your taste buds, and hence palate and brain, alert. Chewing your food slowly and concentrating on its flavors and textures will also increase your sense of satiety, unlike shoveling down a sandwich while you're on the phone to a work colleague, so choose something that you'll really enjoy eating and take time out to savor it. Losing weight is similar to a long-haul journey, so make the trip seem more achievable by breaking it into stages—say morning, afternoon, and evening—and at the end of each stage take a minute to evaluate how you've done. If it's been a good stage, praising yourself will give you the momentum to keep up the good work, but if it's been unsatisfactory, put a lid on it and don't allow feelings of negativity to eat into the following stage. Finally, remember that weight loss is never linear, and you'll inevitably hit a plateau. When this happens, try to stay positive and in control of your eating and exercising, and your weight should soon start to drop off again.

## 10 ways to avoid overeating

1 Drink lots of water while eating to encourage food to swell within your stomach. This stimulates stretch receptors to send messages of satiety to your brain, in turn telling you you've eaten enough.

2 Eat plenty of fresh vegetables and fruits. Besides being chock-full of healthy nutrients, fruits contain slow-release sugars that keep your blood-sugar level stable and encourage your body to produce endorphins, or "happy" hormones. Potatoes apart, have as many vegetables as you like—from artichokes through peas and beans to broccoli and salads—they're all great fiber-providers.

3 Keep your meals simple. Include a small amount of fat, like a little olive oil drizzled over salads and grilled vegetables, but keep your intake of butter, cream and cheese, fatty meats and pâté, pastries, cakes and creamy sauces to a minimum.

4 Eat plenty of lean proteins, such as chicken, fish—both white and oily—and game, eggs, legumes and other vegetable proteins like soy and tofu. Because they make you feel full for some time, proteins are excellent sustainers.

5 Add stomach-satisfying bulk to your meals in the form of root vegetables, like parsnips and carrots, along with pumpkins and squashes. Include small amounts of starchy foods, such as wholewheat bread, pasta, rice, and potatoes. Although some women find that avoiding carbohydrates altogether makes them feel more energetic, I'd instead advise simply eating fewer starchy foods, because low-carb diets drain your body of calcium, while no-carb diets increase your risk of developing heart disease.

6 Have a small cup of excellent coffee after every meal.

7 If you yearn for something sweet, ask yourself why. If it's for comfort, try a healthy alternative like a few fresh or dried fruits (Medjool dates, figs, and mangoes are particularly sweet). If that won't do, have a couple of squares of a chocolate that is rich in cocoa. Sniffing vanilla extract may help, but if all else fails, taking an organic chromium supplement with each meal has been shown to reduce blood-sugar swings.

8 Avoid drinking alcohol on an empty stomach because this will artificially sharpen your appetite.

9 Listen to your body, especially if it's saying you've eaten enough. If it's sending hunger signals, ask yourself if you're genuinely hungry; otherwise comfort or distract yourself with something other than food.

10 Try wearing fewer clothes and turning down the heating to prompt your body to raise its temperature by burning more calories.

# bodyfoods solutions for weight loss

### STRAWBERRY, BANANA, AND RASPBERRY SMOOTHIE (SERVES 2 or 3)

Empty 1 cup strawberries, washed and stalks removed, into a blender with $3/4$ cup raspberries, washed and leaves removed, and 1 large, peeled banana. Blend until smooth. Add 4 Tbs. thick, Greek-style natural yogurt and blend for another minute. Transfer to funky glasses and serve immediately.

### RASPBERRY AND MANGO SALAD (SERVES 4)

First make the raspberry vinaigrette. In the small bowl of your food processor, blend together $3/4$ cup, rounded, fresh raspberries, 2 Tbs. raspberry or red wine vinegar, $1/2$ tsp. Dijon mustard, 1 small garlic clove, 1 tsp. honey, and 5 Tbs. olive oil. Strain through a sieve and discard the seeds. Season with a little sea salt and freshly ground black pepper to taste. When ready to serve, open a bag of ready-made salad of your choice. Empty into a large salad bowl and toss with some of your raspberry vinaigrette. Take a large, ripe mango and cut into slices. Arrange the mango slices over the salad and finish off with a sprinkling of 2 Tbs. pumpkin seeds.

### ZUCCHINI, MINT, TOMATO, AND CORIANDER SEED SALAD (SERVES 4–6)

*If you've ever been on traditional weight-loss diets, you're probably fed up with boring old vegetables, so here's a refreshing salad that won't send the boredom flag flying.*

Soak 1 lb. small, very fresh zucchini in a basin of cold water for about 20 minutes. Cut off the ends, slice the zucchini into small, thin strips, and place the zucchini in a large bowl. Snap the end off 1 firm, green celery stalk and remove the strings. Finely chop another stalk and add it to the zucchini. Now deseed 2 lb. small, ripe, fresh tomatoes. Cut them into bite-sized pieces, and add them to the zucchini mixture, along with 1 finely minced green onion, 2 minced garlic cloves, $1/3$ tsp. crushed coriander seeds and 1 Tbs. chopped fresh mint leaves. Sprinkle some sea salt, the freshly squeezed juice of 1 lemon, 2 Tbs. extra-virgin olive oil, and plenty of freshly ground black pepper on top. Mix the ingredients thoroughly, and place the bowl in the fridge for about 1 hour before serving to enable the flavors to blend and mellow.

## TOMATO AND BASIL SALAD (SERVES 4)

*Making food taste good is a crucial part of losing weight, because the more stimulation the fullness center within your hypothalamus receives, the more quickly you'll feel full. The key to perfecting a good tomato salad is to use ripe tomatoes. To enhance the salad's taste and appearance, try to use a variety of tomatoes of different colors and sizes, such as cherry, plum, yellow-skinned, or green tiger tomatoes.*

You'll need 1 lb. tomatoes of your choice, sliced in half depending on their size. Arrange the tomatoes in a shallow bowl and season with sea salt and freshly ground black pepper. Tear up a generous handful of fresh basil leaves and sprinkle them over the tomatoes, along with 12 roughly chopped, sundried tomatoes preserved in oil (reserve the oil) and 1/4 cup black olives. Meanwhile, make the dressing. Whisk together 3 Tbs. olive oil, 3 Tbs. reserved oil from the sundried tomatoes, 3 Tbs. red wine vinegar, 1 small crushed garlic clove, a pinch of sugar, a little sea salt, and freshly ground black pepper to taste. Pour the dressing over the tomatoes, then sprinkle with 2 very finely minced green onions. Leave the salad to stand at room temperature for 30 minutes to allow the flavors to develop.

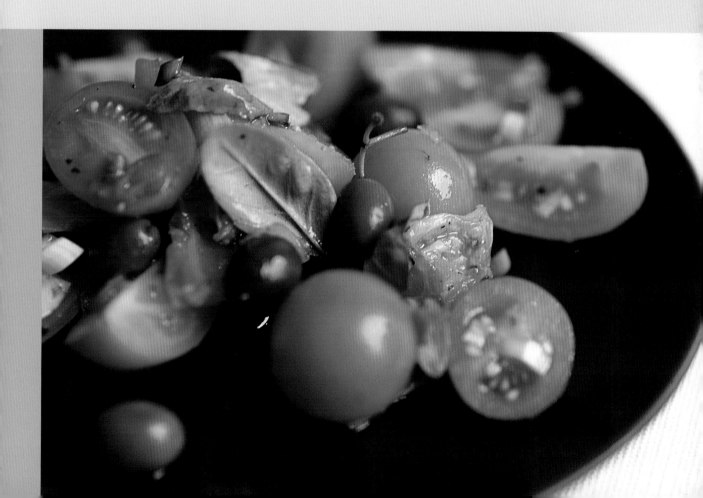

# controlling high and low blood pressure

Although high blood pressure (hypertension) has few symptoms, it can be life threatening, while the symptoms of low blood pressure (hypotension) can be debilitating. Here's how to manage both conditions.

## high blood pressure

Many people don't realize that their stressful lives are taking a toll on their bodies until their doctors diagnose high blood pressure. If left untreated, hypertension—a sign that your circulatory system isn't coping with the pressure you're putting it under—can cause strokes, heart attacks, and kidney conditions, as well as headaches and digestive problems, which is why it should always be treated seriously. Although some people's genetic makeup leaves them susceptible to developing high blood pressure, it is usually linked to lifestyle factors, which means that making certain changes can return it to normal.

Women on the pill, smokers, and older people have an increased risk of developing high blood pressure, as do men. Because stress is a huge contributory factor, the more relaxing activities you can include in your daily life, the more successful you'll be in reducing your blood pressure. Other lifestyle factors that have a big impact on blood pressure are what you eat and drink, and how much. If you're overweight, excess fat presses on the vital blood vessels leading to and from the heart, causing your blood pressure to rise, particularly if you're an apple-shaped person. Losing weight gradually is the answer, but don't crash or yo-yo diet, because these weight-loss strategies will endanger your heart.

It's been shown that blood pressure can be influenced by limiting salt intake, so don't add salt to your cooking or sprinkle it over your food as a matter of course. In fact, weaning yourself off salt enables you to appreciate other flavors far better, especially if you use alternative flavor enhancers, such as lemon, black pepper, garlic, ginger, and other fresh herbs (see pages 20–23). Keep the amount of highly salted foods that you eat to a minimum—notably cured meats like bacon and sausages, pickled foods, olives, salty cheeses, smoked salmon, soy sauce, and other bottled sauces. Boosting your intake of potassium-containing foods is another helpful measure, because potassium depresses sodium (salt) levels within the body. Most fruits and vegetables (especially bananas and tomatoes) contain potassium, as do dried fruits (with no added sulfur dioxide, $SO_2$), legumes, nuts, ginger, and rosemary, so eat plenty of these foods.

Increasing your intake of the omega-3 fatty acids, found in oily fish (like fresh tuna, sardines, salmon, herring, and mackerel), along with eating plenty of seeds, nuts, and garlic, can also help to control hypertension, as can having lots of vitamin E-rich foods, such as vegetable oils, nuts, avocados, fresh fruits, and vegetables. Green, leafy vegetables and dried fruits also offer high levels of calcium, which has been shown to decrease blood pressure. Tread carefully, however, when it comes to the most concentrated calcium sources, namely dairy products, because they contain saturated fats, too, which, if consumed in excess, can raise the body's levels of low-density lipoprotein (LDL), or "bad" cholesterol. Conversely, not only do soy-based foods reduce LDL levels, but recent research has shown that drinking soy milk can significantly lower high blood pressure.

Be warned that regularly overstepping the limits recommended for alcohol consumption (see pages 26–27) will increase your risk of developing high blood pressure, regardless of the antioxidants that alcoholic drinks, and red wine in particular, contain. So restrict yourself to a couple of glasses of your favorite wine a day, ideally for only five days of the week, and enjoy them with a meal, rather than heading straight for the bottle as soon as you walk through the door. On the subject of drinking, downing 5 pints of water a day not only will help your body to absorb the beneficial nutrients from the foods highlighted above but will also encourage it to rid itself of excess sodium.

Finally, it's worth discussing taking Q10, or vitamin Q, with your doctor or dietitian, because this antioxidant seems to have the power to reduce blood pressure. Although we don't yet know how much Q10 the body needs to reap the benefits safely, the consensus seems to be between 100–300mg a day (the most common recommendation being 50mg twice a day) in the form of a supplement, combined with eating more cabbage, brussels sprouts, and broccoli, which appear to stablilize Q10 levels within the body.

## low blood pressure

If your blood pressure tends to be low, you may feel light-headed, particularly after getting up too quickly, have low energy levels, and feel cold and generally weak and wan. And because feeling consistently lousy is no help at all when you're trying to respond to the demands of a busy life, I'd advise trying to raise your blood pressure a little by taking certain dietary measures.

Eating small meals often seems to stave off the symptoms of hypotension, together with snacking on fruits and nuts or wholegrain cookies. The occasional cup of excellent tea or coffee can often give you just the jolt you need to get going, but don't drink too many caffeine-containing drinks, and have plenty of water to limit the caffeine's adverse effects. In contrast to people who suffer from hypertension, including salty foods in your diet can sometimes be a good thing, because it is thought that some instances of hypotension are caused by low adrenal-gland activity, which triggers the body to relinquish sodium. Don't overdose on salty foods, however, because this isn't good for your long-term health. All in all, the better-balanced your diet, the less you should be plagued by the symptoms of low blood pressure.

# bodyfoods solutions for lowering blood pressure

### LIGHT VEGETABLE CASSEROLE (SERVES 6)

*Vegetables are rich in potassium, a mineral that helps to keep blood pressure down. You can almost feel the goodness seeping into you when you eat this fresh, light casserole.*

Slice off the tips of 12 small, tender artichokes, remove the tough, outer leaves (this is vital), and peel the bases. Now cut the artichokes into quarters. If any chokes (inedible centers) have formed, remove them, together with any prickly tips of the inner leaves, then cut each quarter into 3 to create very fine wedges. Place 5–6 sliced green onions and 3 Tbs. water in a heavy-based pan, and cook over a medium heat, stirring constantly, until the water evaporates. Add 4 Tbs. olive oil and sauté the green onions for a few minutes, until they have turned a pale golden color. Add the artichokes, moisten them with a little hot water, and add sea salt to taste. Cover and cook over a low heat for 5 minutes. Now add 2 lb. very young, shelled lima beans and a little more hot water. Cover and cook for another 5 minutes. Add 2 lb. very young, shelled peas, cover and cook for 5 minutes, then sprinkle over 2 Tbs. white wine vinegar and some freshly ground black pepper. Taste and, if necessary, add a little more sea salt. Leave the pan uncovered and cook over a medium-high heat for 2–3 minutes, or until the vinegar has evaporated. Leave to cool, then refrigerate for 24 hours. Serve cold.

### BANANAS AND CUSTARD (SERVES 4)

*A classic! Many of us grew up enjoying this simple, but-now-forgotten combination of bananas and custard sauce or crème anglaise. The quantities below make 1¹/4 cups custard, which can be kept in the fridge for a couple days. If you would like to make the custard foamy, whisk up the egg whites and gently fold them into the prepared custard just before serving.*

Pour 1¹/4 cups whole milk into a pan and drop in 1 split vanilla bean. Bring the milk to the boil, then switch off the heat and leave the vanilla to infuse the milk with its delicious flavor. After about 10 minutes, remove the pod and stir in 1 Tbs. fine granulated sugar. Separate 2 medium eggs, setting aside the whites. Stir a little of the hot milk into the egg yolks. Now pour the egg-yolk mixture into the remaining milk and return it to the heat, stirring constantly until the custard has thickened to a smooth, saucelike consistency. Serve with slices of ripe banana.

## *herbal first aid for hypertension*

The following essential oils can combat high blood pressure: clary sage, lavender, and marjoram.

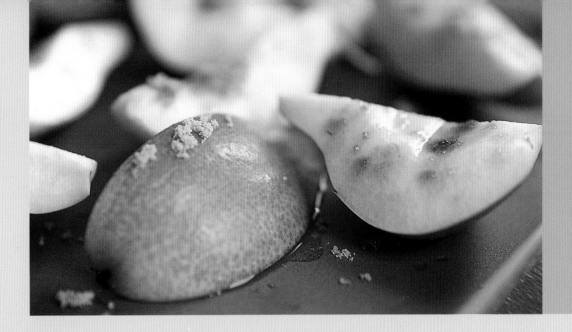

## TRAY-BAKED PEARS WITH ROASTED HAZELNUTS (SERVES 2)

*Fruits contain slow-release sugars, which help ease fatigue. Since sometimes a tired gut can be overly sensitive to raw fruits, I've cooked these pears to make them easy to digest and more satisfying. Cooked fruits make a fantastic dessert all year round, be they soft, ripe peaches popped onto a barbecue in the summer or apples baked in the oven and sprinkled with roasted nuts in the fall.*

Heat the oven to 425°. Then cut 2 evenly sized pears, such as Barlett or Bosc, into quarters, also cutting off the stalks and removing the cores. Scatter the pear pieces over a roasting tray and sprinkle over 1 Tbs. granulated brown sugar and a splash of your favorite alcohol, perhaps brandy or Calvados. Bake for 5–6 minutes, or until the pears are tender and light golden in color. Meanwhile, place a scant 1/4 cup hazelnuts on another small baking tray, and pop it into the oven for 2–3 minutes, or until the hazelnuts are lightly roasted. When you are ready to serve the pears, simply sprinkle some of the cracked, roasted hazelnuts on top; perhaps serve with a dollop of Greek-style natural yogurt.

## KUMQUATS DIPPED IN DARK CHOCOLATE (SERVES 1)

*Excess weight around the middle aggravates blood pressure, which means you need a small and satisfying dessert that won't pile on the pounds. These chocolate-dipped kumquats should fit the bill. They're so delicious that you'll feel relaxed just as soon as you pop one in your mouth! Eat the entire fruit, the skin as well as the flesh (but spit out the pips). Its hints of orange, lime, and bergamot complement the chocolate perfectly.*

Wash 4 oz. kumquats. In a pan, melt a 3 oz. bar of good-quality (minimum 70% cocoa solids), dark chocolate, and simply dip the kumquats into it.

# attacking high cholesterol levels

Cholesterol is manufactured mainly by the liver. It is circulated within the blood and is vital for the body's efficient functioning, particularly in terms of producing sex hormones such as testosterone. The amount of cholesterol generated by your liver is influenced by several factors, including your genes, your stress level, and how much fat, especially saturated animal fat, you consume.

There are two main types of cholesterol: one "bad", namely low-density lipoprotein (LDL), and one "good", namely high-density lipoprotein (HDL). LDL is labeled "bad" because if there is too much of it circulating in the blood, it tends to be deposited in the blood vessels, causing them to fur up, which can lead to heart disease and strokes. By contrast, HDL earns its "good" tag by helping to pick up and remove LDL from the body via the gut. If you are diagnosed as having a high LDL level, it is vital that you watch what you eat and drink. The following tips will help you keep within the healthy limits.

## eat to beat cholesterol

Eat as many antioxidant-rich foods as you can, because the nutrients—including vitamin C, beta carotene, vitamin E, and selenium—in dried and fresh fruits and vegetables help to prevent LDL from being deposited in the blood vessels. Specifically:

Pineapple, rich in bromelain, which is thought to clear blocked arteries and thin the blood, thus fighting off heart disease and strokes. It also aids digestion.

The allium family of vegetables, which includes onions, leeks, garlic, and chives, provides us with organo-sulfides which boost the immune system, fight cancers, help to prevent heart disease, and encourage stomach ulcers to heal. Garlic is rich in allicin, too, which has long been renowned for its antibacterial, antiviral properties and its ability to lower LDL and increase "good" HDL levels.

Quercetin, an antioxidant found in red wine, black and green tea, apples, tomatoes, potatoes, and grapes, is believed to ward off heart disease, cataracts, and hay fever. Green tea is one of its richest providers (it's best not to add milk, though, because this neutralizes its antioxidant power).

Prunes, strawberries, apples, citrus fruits, raisins, raspberries, blackberries, walnuts, and pecans are rich in other flavonoids, as are dark chocolate, red wine, and beans, including soy beans.

Capsaicin, found in chilies, can lower "bad", LDL cholestrol levels, also averting heart disease through its powerful antioxidant properties and reducing inflammation.

Vegetables and fruits contain coumarins, but licorice offers the highest concentration of this nutrient, which is believed to thin the blood, thus preventing strokes and heart disease.

Boost your intake of oily fish, such as salmon, mackerel, sardines, herrings, and fresh tuna, because their omega-3 fatty acids prevent LDL from being deposited in the blood vessels and blood clots from forming.

- Eat the foods that produce HDL, particularly oily fish, garlic, fruits and vegetables, fiber and wholegrains.
- Increase your intake of soluble fiber, found in oats, legumes, fruits, and vegetables.
- Drink 5 pints of water a day to encourage the fiber in food to swell in your stomach, stimulating the liver to produce HDL, as well as cushioning the rate and level at which your body absorbs fat.
- Include some soy-based products (such as soy yogurt and milk) in your diet, because soy is believed to reduce the risk of heart disease and strokes.

## some more anti-LDL tips

Don't eat too many saturated animal fats (like dairy products and fatty meat), which encourage the liver to manufacture LDL; but when you do, team them with water and a fiber-containing food (enjoy a slice of cheese with wholewheat bread and a glass of water, for example). On the subject of cheese, cutting the rind off soft cheeses dramatically reduces their fat content. When it comes to hard cheeses, use a cheese slice rather than hacking off a big chunk. If the flavor of the cheese is enhanced, you tend to eat less of it, so choose a sharp cheese over a mild one, and when cooking with cheese, try adding a little mustard. An increased consumption of monounsaturated fats (as typified by a Mediterranean diet) is linked with a lower risk of developing heart disease and certain cancers, so eat lots of foods that offer them, including olive oil, macadamia nuts, almonds, canola oil, and hazelnuts. Peanuts are quite high in monounsaturated fats, too, so a few plain peanuts (not salted or dry-roasted ones) or peanut butter (with a high peanut content) spread over wholewheat bread makes a good snack.

Keep your intake of vitamin E-rich foods high, because their d-alpha tocopherol, a powerful antioxidant, has been shown to play a crucial role in protecting blood vessels from the buildup of LDL. A supplement doesn't have the same effect, so it's best to focus on dietary sources of vitamin E, including vegetable oils (such as olive and sunflower oil), nuts, sundried tomatoes, avocados (spread guacamole over your sandwich rather than butter), whole grains and even plain, homemade popcorn. Don't consume too many of these foods if you're on Warfarin or other blood-thinning drugs, however, because vitamin E tends to thin blood, too. Because regular exercise lowers both stress and LDL levels, keep fit!

## some more HDL-promoting tips

Reduce your intake of the foods that can lower the body's level of HDL, particularly processed foods containing trans-fatty acids, hard margarines, and cooking fats (other than olive oil). Apart from canola oil, vegetable oils like sunflower oil are relatively high in the polyunsaturated fats that can produce trans-fatty acids when heated, so stick to using olive oil, poured straight from the bottle. Drink a couple of glasses of antioxidant-rich wine or beer a day to encourage your body to produce HDL. Not only that, but their anthrocyanins and other antioxidants can prevent LDL from being deposited in your blood vessels.

# bodyfoods solutions for preventing heart disease

### PINEAPPLE AND MACADAMIA BULGING OAT MUFFINS (MAKES 6)

*Muffins are unbelievably fast to make, as you just mix everything together. They will probably not hang around too long, either, as they are fantastic eaten while still warm.*

Heat the oven to 400°. Place 6 paper muffin cups in a muffin tray. Mix together in a large bowl 3/4 cup whole-wheat flour, 1 tsp. baking powder and 1/2 cup rolled oats. In a pitcher mix together 1 large beaten egg, 1/4 cup granulated brown sugar, a generous 1/2 cup milk and 4 Tbs. melted butter. Make a well in the center of the dry ingredients and pour in the wet ingredients. Fold in very gently, then carefully stir in 5/8 cup chopped, ready-to-eat pineapple chunks. Divide the mixture between the paper cups, then sprinkle with 1 Tbs. finely chopped macadamia nuts. Bake in the oven for 20 minutes until risen and golden. Transfer to a wire rack to cool.

### ROASTED VEGETABLE SOUP (SERVES 4)

*This is a great recipe, as it is packed full of fresh vegetables, which are roasted together with garlic and rosemary. Not much oil has been added, so it is very low in fat. If you have your own fresh stock that's ideal; otherwise try to buy a good-quality stock, as it will make all the difference.*

Heat the oven to 400°. Peel and roughly chop into chunks 2 large carrots, 2 large parsnips, 2 red onions, and 2 large sweet potatoes, and roughly chop 1 large leek and 2 large red bell peppers. Spread them in a large roasting tin and drizzle over 1 Tbs. olive oil on top; add 3 whole garlic cloves, 2 sprigs rosemary, and plenty of seasoning. Give the pan a good shake to coat everything in the oil, then put in the oven to roast for 45 minutes, or until slightly charred and tender. Remove half the vegetables and set aside. Then transfer the remainder to a food processor and pour in a generous 2 pints of vegetable stock. Process until smooth, then pour into a large pan and add the reserved vegetables. Heat through and season to taste. When ready to serve, ladle into bowls and serve with some chunky brown bread.

## ROASTED COD SALAD WITH A HORSERADISH CREAM DRESSING (SERVES 2)

*Horseradish is a traditional accompaniment to beef, but since too much red meat is bad for our hearts, I've used it with cod, a fish that is very low in saturated animal fat. The horseradish dressing that accompanies this salad, which serves two, is both piquant and a refreshing contrast to the warm roasted cod and tomatoes. It would also be fabulous with smoked fish.*

Heat the oven to 425°. In a shallow roasting pan, mix together 1 small crushed garlic clove, 1 Tbs. chopped fresh parsley, and 2 Tbs. olive oil. Season well with freshly ground black pepper and sea salt, then rub the oil all over two 5 oz. thick cod fillets. Place the roasting tray in the oven for 10 minutes, or until the cod is cooked, adding 2 lengths of vine-ripened cherry tomatoes after 5 minutes. Meanwhile, make the dressing by mixing together a generous $5/8$ cup sour cream, 2 tsp. creamed horseradish, and 2 tsp. capers. Season to taste, then set the dressing aside. When you're ready to serve the salad, arrange a few watercress and arugula leaves on each of two serving plates. Top with the roasted cod and tomatoes, then drizzle the horseradish dressing on top. Serve immediately.

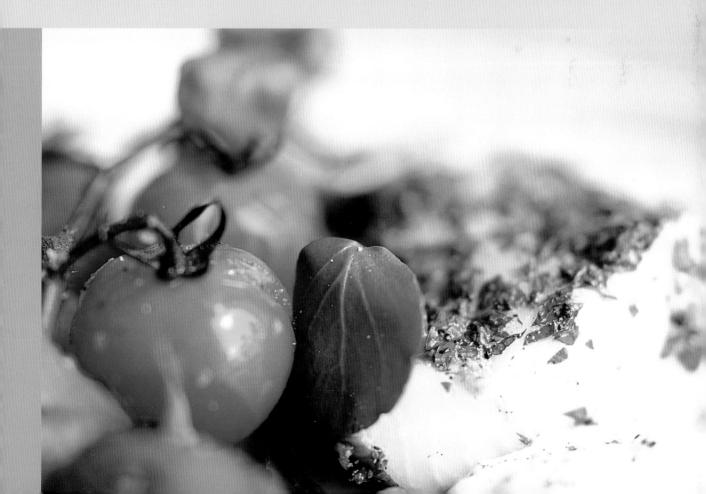

# reducing the risk
# of cancer

Experts believe that as many as 30–40 percent of cancers in the West are connected with diet, which makes it more than worth your while looking at how, and what, you eat and drink, along with your lifestyle.

Diet apart, besides giving up smoking, try to keep your weight within the ideal range, because being overweight is linked with cancer of the breast, gall bladder, and prostate. And if you're tempted to cut nutritional corners and take a supplement, I'd urge you not to, because some have been shown actually to increase the risk of succumbing to certain cancers. Beta carotene, for instance, when taken by smokers, was shown to increase their susceptibility to lung cancer. Food, like life, should be enjoyed, so try to regard eating as a self-nurturing pleasure rather than a medical regime. When it comes to your diet, there are ten vital elements you should try to incorporate to reduce your risk of developing cancer, as well as to fight it if it has already struck.

## 10 preventive measures to stay cancer-free

1 Build up a strong antioxidant presence in your body to help to neutralize the dangerous free radicals that the body produces in response to radiation and certain toxins. The most effective antioxidants in this respect are offered by foods that are rich in vitamin A (such as oily fish, meat, and dairy products) and beta carotene (which is converted into vitamin A within the body and is found mostly in red, orange, and yellow fruits and vegetables), vitamin C (which all fruits and vegetables contain), vitamin E (the richest sources are vegetables and vegetable oils, nuts, avocados, and whole-wheat cereals), vitamin D (oily fish is an excellent source), vitamin K (found in dark green, leafy vegetables, fruit, and vegetable skins) and certain of the B vitamins (which many foods, but primarily whole grains, contain).

2 The selenium that nuts (particularly brazil nuts), seeds (notably flaxseeds), tuna fish, fruits, and vegetables contain is another powerful ally in the battle against cancer, as is the isoflavone soy (so think about switching to soy milk and yogurt, and try my soy shake on page 39), black currants, elderberries, and green tea. The leading isoflavone is genistein (which you can take as a daily supplement of 40–50mg).

3 Stimulate your body to produce higher levels of detoxifying enzymes (which can both reduce the damaging effects of free radicals and encourage the body to rid itself of carcinogens) by eating foods that contain sulforophane and quercetin. These nutrients are found in broccoli, cabbage, red bell peppers, peas, rosemary, and basil (so think along the lines of a fresh pesto, tomato, and basil salad), leeks, citrus fruits, and onions.

4 Incorporate foods into your diet that help to shield the body's cells against harmful agents. Among the most powerful are those that contain flavonoids (citrus fruits, grapes, and wine—grapes also providing ellagic acid, another cancer-blocker, as do strawberries and cherries) and immuno-enhancers. Immuno-enhancers, which boost the immune system's ability to defend the body against cancer cells, include such herbs as echinacea (which increases the body's army of natural killer cells and encourages it to produce interferon, a natural, anti-carcinogenic "hormone") and fibrous foods.

5 Eat as much organic produce as possible, because it appears to offer higher levels of such cancer-inhibiting nutrients as flavonoids than do nonorganic foods.

6 Lactobacilli and bifido bacteria, the cultures present in live yogurt, have been shown to improve the immune system's performance, so focus on eating these "good" bacteria in the form of live yogurt (perhaps mixed with fruits) and seeds, as either a light breakfast or a snack. Increasing the amount of prebiotic foods or promoters of such "good" bacteria (artichokes, Belgian endive, oats, and onions) in your diet will also help to nurture a healthy bacterial balance within your gut.

7 If you've been diagnosed with cancer, eating fresh, carotenoid-rich foods (namely red and orange fruits and vegetables like oranges, carrots, red bell peppers, and tomatoes) and dark green, leafy vegetables (such as spinach and broccoli) can help to control the cancer cells' activity. The carotenoid found in tomatoes and its products, such as tomato paste and ketchup, is lycopene; to maximize the amount of lycopene that your body gleans, choose dark red tomatoes, which have the highest lycopene content, and fry them in olive oil to make it more accessible to the body. Other redifferentiators, as such compounds are called, include the resveratrol found in wine and the butyrate (a fatty acid) that bifido bacteria (see 6, above) produce within the gut.

8 Concentrate on eating as many oily fish, seeds, and nuts as you can, all of which are rich in beneficial polyunsaturated omega oils, but limit your consumption of saturated fats like fatty and red meat and dairy products, because a high intake can increase your risk of developing colon cancer.

9 Rather than roasting and broiling foods, try to steam, poach, or boil them. This may not be an appetizing option when it comes to cooking high-protein foods such as fish, chicken, and meat, but at least try to steam—or even microwave—vegetables. The problem with exposing food to a high heat or naked flame is that it produces carcinogens as it browns. And because reheating oil has a similar effect, use a vegetable oil—ideally olive oil—when frying, and use it only once. Don't eat too many cured products, such as salami and smoked meat and fish, and also limit your intake of pickles.

10 Drink alcohol only in moderation, because an excessive intake increases your vulnerability to several cancers. Red wine appears to be the most healthful option, but still don't imbibe too much.

# bodyfoods solutions for preventing cancer

### BAKED BEET AND APPLE SALAD (SERVES 2)

*Fresh beets taste fabulous when baked, because baking both brings out their natural sweetness and intensifies their flavor. A word of caution: don't wear white when making this salad!*

Heat the oven to 400°. Wash and scrub 2 medium-sized beets, then wrap each in a piece of aluminum foil and place them on a baking tray. Bake in the oven for 35–40 minutes, or until the beetroots are tender. Meanwhile, make a chive vinaigrette by whisking together 2 Tbs. finely snipped fresh chives, 1 Tbs. white wine vinegar, and 3 Tbs. light olive oil. Season to taste with freshly ground black pepper and sea salt, and set aside. Heat 1 Tbs. olive oil in a skillet and fry 1 red onion, sliced into rings, until it is light brown in color and crisp. Spoon the onion rings onto a paper towel and leave them to drain and cool. Add 1 Tbs. olive oil to the skillet and fry 1 eating apple, cut into thick wedges, until it is golden. When the beets are cool enough to handle, remove them from the foil and cut them into thick wedges. Just before serving, place a few spinach and watercress leaves on each plate, and then scatter the beet and apple wedges on top. Drizzle the chive vinaigrette on top, sprinkle with the crisp onion rings, and serve immediately.

### BITTER LEAF HERB SALAD WITH MAPLE MUSTARD DRESSING (SERVES 6)

Empty a large bag of ready-to-use mixed bitter salad greens into a large serving bowl. Add a couple of handfuls of mixed torn herbs (basil, mint, tarragon, parsley) and mix through the leaves. Meanwhile, make the dressing: whisk together in a small pitcher 3 Tbs. olive oil, 2 Tbs. whole-grain mustard, 1 Tbs. maple syrup, 1 tsp. white wine vinegar, and plenty of seasoning to taste. When you are ready to serve, pour over enough dressing to lightly coat the leaves, then, if you like, sprinkle a handful of spiced roasted nuts and seeds on top.

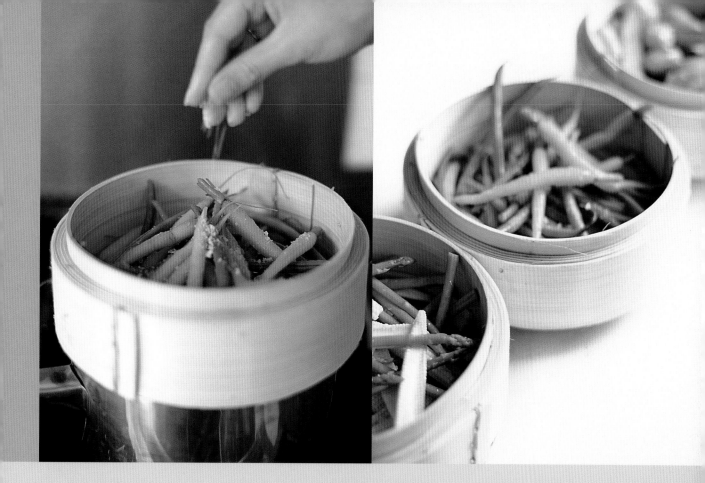

## STEAMED BABY VEGETABLES (SERVES 4)

*With this recipe you must be very open-minded and use the vegetables you like or are able to source. Steaming is a perfect way to cook vegetables to get them to that just al dente texture. Instead of investing in a rather expensive steamer, why not measure your largest pan and find a cheap Chinese bamboo steamer that will fit on top and do the job just as well.*

Bring a large pan of salted water to the boil and add 9 oz. baby new potatoes. Leave to simmer for 12–15 minutes until just tender. Meanwhile, position the steamer on top of the pan and after about 8 minutes of the potatoes' cooking, add 9 oz. baby carrots in the bottom section of the steamer, then cover with the lid. After about 3 minutes, add 9 oz. baby zucchini. Place the next basket layer of the steamer over the carrots and zucchini, then add 1 scant cup baby sweetcorn, 1 scant cup asparagus tips, and 1½ cups fine green beans, trimmed and cut in two. Cover again and leave to steam for 2–3 minutes. When ready to serve, transfer the vegetables to a warmed serving dish. Drizzle a little olive oil and a squeeze of lemon juice on top. Sprinkle some sea salt and a good grinding of black pepper on top, then serve immediately.

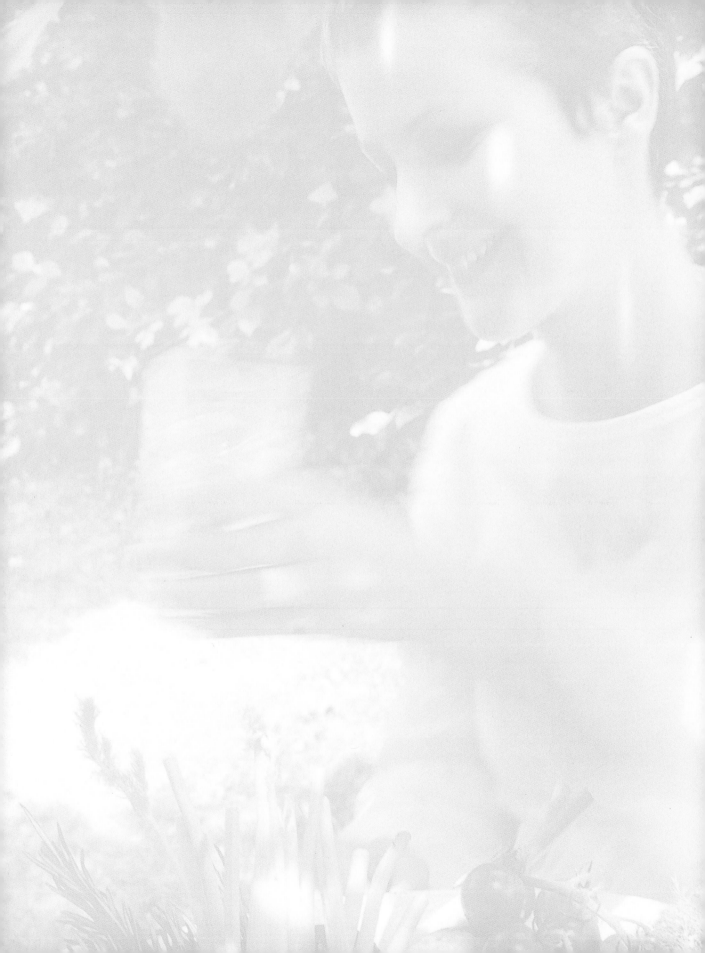

# bodyfoods
# stress-busters

Feeling overly anxious, or panicky, is usually due to an overload of stress, causing your body to produce a flood of epinephrine—the "fight or flight" hormone— to deal with the situation. This condition doesn't occur only when you're facing a crisis, however, but may become the norm if you're constantly feeling under pressure and stressed, so that the smallest upset can trigger your heart to race, causing palpitations, and making you feel panic-stricken, sweaty, nauseous, dizzy, and generally out of control. If this description fits you, I'd advise you to seek professional help to try to work out what's underlying your chronic state of anxiety, but you can also help yourself by eating the nutrients that best calm body and mind.

# combating the symptoms of stress

As a previous sufferer of panic attacks, I have delved deep into the archives to try to discover how food and drink can help us avoid having them, or at least cope with them when they do strike.

## stress symptoms checklist

When I'm starting to feel increasingly anxious, I run through the following checklist to try to work out whether I'm suffering from a stress overload.

- Am I eating more or less than usual? (I find that being under extreme stress usually puts me off my food.)
- Am I beginning to sleep particularly badly, tossing and turning throughout the night and then waking up early feeling drained?
- Am I losing my sense of humor and looking at things in an overly pessimistic light?
- Am I becoming so irritated that I tend to snap when the smallest things go wrong?
- Do tiny upsets make me burst into tears, especially at inopportune moments and in inappropriate places? (Although I find crying a release, it's often a response to great stress, which isn't good in itself.)

## stress-busting solutions

If running through my checklist sets alarm bells ringing, I immediately take the following steps. But even if your stress levels don't trigger anxiety attacks, everyone agrees that the better you look after your body, the less likely it is that stress will drag you down.

- I make sure that plenty of healthful foods and ingredients for proper meals are on hand by restocking my pantry, refrigerator and freezer (see pages 46–51). If I'm out and about, I supply myself with energizing snacks (see pages 58–9) to ensure that I don't deprive my body of vital nutrients by not eating well.
- Because eating in company when under stress doesn't bode well for the digestive system (which is particularly sensitive to feelings of anxiety), I cancel any business lunches.
- I pencil in time for myself in my diary, retreat into my shell, and turn off the phone. My needs are currently greater than anyone else's.
- I make sure that I spend at least two quiet evenings relaxing at home.
- I focus on doing breathing and relaxation exercises (see pages 140, 148, and 154–5) and use the kidney massage technique described on page 155.
- I book a massage or facial or simply soak in a warm bath, to which I've added either some soothing essential oils or Epsom salts, which aid relaxation by encouraging the body to relinquish its toxins and the mind its feelings of stress. I also burn some calming essential oils, such as lavender and rose.
- I sprinkle a few drops of lavender essential oil over my pillow to help me to sleep and then go to bed early.

## cut out the caffeine

Above all, avoid caffeine-containing drinks and foods like coffee, tea, cola, and chocolate, which are major anxiety-aggravators. Not only does caffeine act as an unwanted stimulant, making you feel even more wired, it keeps you awake at night, leaving you feeling exhausted the next day and exaggerating your feelings of anxiety. Instead of coffee or tea, turn to either calming herbal teas like camomile, lemon verbena, and vervain (see page 13) or plain water. All of these both soothe you and help you to stay sufficiently alert to deal with the demands of a busy day.

Another of caffeine's effects is feeling as though your blood-sugar level has dropped through the floor and consequently making you weak, light-headed, and even more anxious. This triggers the body to generate epinephrine with which to release emergency supplies of sugar from its glycogen stores in an attempt to compensate. My first full-blown panic attack occurred when I was dehydrated, overtired, and had drunk a strong cup of coffee. The final straw was when I then accepted a sugar-loaded cookie because the sugar was rapidly absorbed into my bloodstream, sending my blood-sugar level shooting up and then crashing down again, forcing my body to generate yet more epinephrine. Panic ensued. Ever since, I've avoided eating foods that contain rapidly absorbed sugars on an empty stomach, and if I need a sweet fix, I opt for fruit rather than chocolate or cookies.

## avoid aggravating alcohol

If you're prone to feeling stressed, be warned that although it's fine to unwind with the occasional glass of wine, trying to relieve your anxiety by hitting the bottle places you in danger of crossing the threshold from anxiety to panic. It's also best to get into the habit of having small, well-balanced meals to keep your blood-sugar level constant without overwhelming your body with a large amount of food, which prompts blood to be diverted to the stomach to aid digestion, sometimes causing palpitations. And because the body seems to use up its supply of B vitamins faster than usual when under stress, focus on eating foods that are rich in these nutrients (including whole grains, all types of fish, lean protein, seeds, nuts, and cheese).

## herbal first aid for alleviating stress

Add a few drops of Bach's Five-flower Rescue Remedy (something I always carry with me) or Bach's Mimulus Original Flower Remedy to a glass of water and then sip it slowly.

Use stress-busting homeopathic remedies like Aconite, Nux vomica, or Arg-nit.

# stress-busting bodyfoods

## MUSHROOM RISOTTO (SERVES 4–6)

*Risotto may seem a cumbersome meal to make, but if you have the energy to stand for 20 minutes, you should find that the monotonous action of stirring acts as a hypnotic stress buster. Rice also seems to encourage the body to produce soporific hormones to wind us down rather than up!*

1 cup dried mushrooms

a generous 2 pints chicken stock

2 Tbs. olive oil

2 Tbs. unsalted butter

2 shallots, peeled and minced

Carnaroli or Arborio rice

1/4 cup Parmesan cheese, freshly grated

Soak the mushrooms in 2 cups warm water for 30 minutes or until the water has turned dark. Strain the mushrooms through a sieve lined with a paper towel to remove any dirt, saving the water. Rinse the mushrooms in fresh water until they are very clean. In a saucepan, heat the stock until it is simmering slowly and steadily. Add the olive oil and half the butter to a heavy-bottomed sauce pan and sauté the shallots until soft, but not brown. Add the rice, stirring until the grains are well coated, and cook for a couple of minutes to warm them through. Now add the stock, a ladle at a time, allowing the rice to soak up all of the liquid before adding another ladle. After about 10 minutes, add the reserved mushroom water, again a ladle at a time, until it is used up. Now add the mushrooms, stirring gently as you continue to add the stock, until the rice is cooked, but not mushy—it should retain some texture. When the rice is cooked, turn off the heat and add the Parmesan and remaining butter. Now check the seasoning; you shouldn't need to add much sea salt because the stock is likely to have been quite salty, but sprinkle plenty of black pepper over the risotto, then serve it immediately.

## SIMPLE GARLIC AND FRESH HERB PASTA (SERVES 2)

*If you get home stressed and late from work and need to unwind quickly and easily, make this combination of pasta (which encourages our bodies to relax), herbs, and good-quality olive oil; it takes only as long to make as the pasta takes to boil.*

Bring a pan of salted water to the boil, drop in 4 oz. dried tagliatelle (or other pasta) and cook according to the instructions on the package. (I think dried pasta gives the best, non-mushy results, and you can keep it in your kitchen cabinet for months.) Meanwhile, in a serving bowl, mix together 1 tsp. freshly grated lemon zest, the freshly squeezed juice of 1/2 lemon, 1 tsp. finely chopped capers, 1 small pinch chili flakes, 1 small crushed garlic clove, 2 Tbs. freshly chopped parsley, and 2 Tbs. extra-virgin olive oil. Season well with freshly ground black pepper and sea salt. Drain the pasta and add it to the flavored oil,

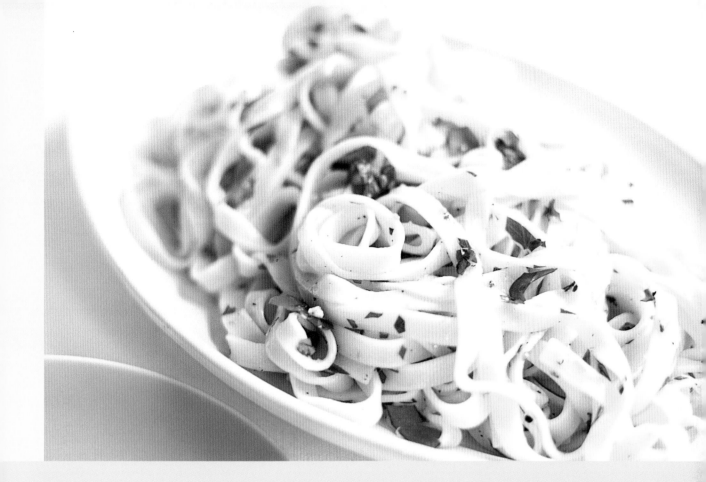

tossing it thoroughly to ensure that the oil is evenly distributed. Top with shavings of fresh Parmesan cheese and tuck in at once.

## STRAWBERRY AND PASSION FRUIT YOGURT FOOL (SERVES 2)

*A "fool" is a traditional English dessert made of puréed fruit and cream or custard. This yogurt version is delectable!*

Place 6 heaped Tbs. Greek-style, natural yogurt, the juice of 1 orange, and the seeds of 1 passion fruit in a small bowl, and gently combine them until the mixture is well blended. Slice about 10 large, ripe strawberries into quarters, and reserve 8 quarters for decoration. Place the remaining quarters in a small bowl and sprinkle them with a little black pepper to enhance their flavor. Mash the strawberries with a fork until they are soft, but retain some texture, and then combine them with the yogurt mixture. Divide the fool between two small serving dishes and arrange the reserved strawberry quarters on top.

## WARM MILK WITH DATES (SERVES 1)

Three-quarters fill a large mug with low-fat milk. Place a date in the milk, then pop the mug into the microwave. Heat up and then allow to cool, then remove the date. Drink right away for a destressing evening drink.

# stress-busting workout

However busy my life becomes, I've found that exercise is something that I simply can't skip. Not only does it keep me fit, but I've found it one of the best stress busters of all, because it stimulates the brain to produce endorphins, the "happy hormones" that lift your mood and give you the energy and motivation to keep going. When stress is really getting to me, exercise sharpens up my fuzzy brain, giving me clarity of thought and focus, and uses up the surplus epinephrine that floods my body when I'm under pressure.

The best type of exercise to take depends on what you want to achieve. If losing weight and improving the health of your heart are your aims, then aerobic exercises like swimming, running, cycling, walking briskly, and skipping rope are the ones for you. Alternatively, if you want to improve your musculature and tone your body, physiologists recommend anaerobic exercises such as light weight-training, pilates, yoga, and resistance exercises. Both types improve how your body moves and looks, and how positive you feel about it as a result, as well as the minimizing effect that stress has on you. (The exercises on pages 140, 148 and 154 work wonders in this respect.)

I find swimming particularly healing; the cool water caressing my body seems to wash away my worries, while concentrating on nothing more than performing the strokes has the same effect on me as meditation. When I'm all exercised out, I find a combination of essential oils (see page 154) and basking in the warmth of a sauna a fantastic way of unwinding and detoxifying my body (but check with your doctor before using a sauna if you suffer from any medical condition).

## schedule your exercise sessions

Whatever type of exercise you settle on, do as I do: plan ahead and pencil exercise sessions into your desk calender as though they were meetings. Otherwise you'll find that the week is eaten away by other things, so that by the end of it your good intentions will have come to naught. You'll feel so much fitter and brimming with energy if you exercise regularly—for at least 20–30 minutes three times a week—that you'll recoup the working time you worried about losing by being able to perform both more intensively and faster.

If your life is so frenetic that you can't afford the time to go to the gym (and when you're time-poor, traveling there and back, changing and showering, quite apart from exercising, can be too much of a hassle), why not exercise at home? There are lots of great exercise videos and DVDs on the market, as well as exercise machines (although because they're expensive, and the chances are that yours may end up sitting idle after a few sessions, I'd either try to build up a regular exercise routine before investing in one or else buy a secondhand machine). Other alternatives include walking to work, taking a brisk stroll at lunchtime or getting off the bus a few stops before your destination and then walking the rest of the way—what could be easier, or cheaper? Indeed, you needn't spend a fortune on equipment when all you need is a good pair of running shoes (and how about a jump rope?).

## eating for exercise

If you're to reap the rewards of exercise, however, it's important to eat the right things at the right times. It's best not to exercise when you're either ravenously hungry and feeling shaky due to a low blood-sugar level (in which case you may pass out) or when you've just eaten a meal.

If you prefer to exercise first thing in the morning, the solution is to have a snack, such as a banana or small tub of yogurt, before exercising and breakfast afterward. Similarly, if you're an evening exerciser, have a substantial late-afternoon snack—perhaps a whole-wheat sandwich or some oat crackers and a few sustaining fruits like bananas or dried figs, or else a slice of whole-wheat bread spread with pure-fruit jam or a bowl of soup—a couple of hours before working out and a small, light meal like a simple pasta dish or a baked potato afterward. And while you're actually exercising, remember to keep your body hydrated by taking small sips of water from a bottle (don't waste your money on "sports" drinks unless you're a very dedicated athlete).

## how strenuous?

One question that I'm frequently asked is how hard does exercise need to be in order to be effective? Well, your heart should ideally be performing at 60–80 percent of your maximum heart rate for your age, and a simple equation can help you to work this out. The equation is as follows: subtract your age from 220 to find your maximum heart rate, then calculate 60–80 percent of this figure to give you the number of heartbeats per minute to aim for when exercising. Check this by taking your pulse every so often the first few times you work out to assess how strenuously you need to exercise and also how your body's feeling as a result—the easiest way to do this is to press your fingers to each side of your neck until you can feel your pulse and count the number of heartbeats over 10 seconds, then multiply that number by 6 to get your heartbeats per minute. You shouldn't be seriously out of breath or feel sick, nor should you feel as though you're under-exercising. Remember that pushing your heart rate above your ideal zone is pointless, especially if you're trying to lose weight, because this has an anaerobic effect that forces your body to burn sugar (not fat) and to produce substances called ketones, which make you feel sick, give you cramps, and generally aren't the least bit beneficial to your health.

# stress-management techniques

For the past ten years, I've worked alongside Dr. Katingo Giannoulis, a consultant clinical psychologist who has helped many of my clients work through their psychological problems (which often include issues related to living in today's stressful environment) in a very empowering and practical way. So that you, too, can benefit from her wisdom, here are some of Katingo's ideas on how best to manage stress.

Some stress is necessary for normal functioning because the nervous system needs some stimulation if it is to function well. Moderate levels of stress are therefore useful. When stress is either too low or too high, however, people perform a task less well. Stress is a problem only when it occurs too often, too intensely, for too long, and in the wrong situation. Stress is not something tangible, but how we interpret what is happening around us. As Shakespeare wisely wrote in *Hamlet*, "There is nothing either good or bad, but thinking makes it so."

Before beginning to learn ways of managing your stress, it is worth attempting to monitor it by keeping a stress diary, specifying the situations or triggers that led up to the stress and your resultant emotions and thoughts. This will help you to identify common triggers and may also enable you to anticipate potentially stressful situations.

## 3 ways to manage stress effectively

You will find that the most effective way of managing stress is to adopt a three-pronged approach. Combine the strategies suggested here to change the way your body reacts, the way you think, and the way you behave when under stress.

### 1 change your bodily reactions

The following stategies will change the way your body reacts to stress and give you a sense of control and well-being:

- relaxation training, yoga, or meditation
- controlled breathing (for instance, counting backward from 100 to 1 in threes, or counting forward from 1 to 100 in sevens, while controlling your breathing rate)
- visualization or picturing (athletes often use this strategy before a competition by visualizing themselves performing really well and winning)
- regular exercise
- aromatherapy or massage

## 2 change your negative thinking

In order to cope with the negative thinking that typically accompanies stress, firstly try to identify where the stress stems from (a potential change like moving, for instance, or the stress of potential failure or criticism). Your stress diary will help you to do this. Now try to use some "mental first aid" or quick stress-control techniques that enable you to deal with the specific stress there and then. Remember that what you feel is the result of what you think, and your self-talk will determine how you react in stressful situations.

- Distract yourself from the stress by focusing on your environment or reciting multiplication tables, poetry, or song lyrics in your mind.
- Try using mental imagery to cope with sudden stress. For example, generate a mental picture of relaxation, perhaps snow-capped mountains or a seascape, to which you can refer whenever you feel stressed. Keep referring to that picture in your mind until the stress reaction begins to dissipate.
- If appropriate, it may sometimes be worth trying to ridicule the worry.
- Think about the worst thing that could possibly happen and generate a solution for such a scenario.
- Detach yourself from the situation by imagining how someone you respect would cope with the problem.

## 3 change any stress-related behavior

The following ideas will help you to change stress-related behavior such as avoidance, aggression, comfort-eating or drinking, smoking, or drug use:

- Learn the value of prioritization. This is the very essence of good time management, good organization skills, and realistic goal setting. If the stress is to do with poor time management, you'll find it useful to monitor how you use your time with the help of a diary.
- Recognize the importance and use of support.
- Rehearse how to cope with stressful situations that you can predict (such as a job interview), ideally with support so that you can be given constructive feedback.
- Introduce "active" relaxing situations in your life (like going for walks in the park; having warm, aromatic, candlelit baths to relaxing music; allowing yourself to be pampered occasionally; or spending some time at an art exhibition without putting yourself under time pressure). Sitting in front of the television and drinking or eating is a "passive" form of relaxation that often does not relax us at all.
- Avoid avoidance. The more you avoid a stress-inducing situation, the more you will be unable to cope and consequently the more you will need to continue to rely on avoidance as a way of getting by. If there are certain stress-producing situations that you tend to avoid (social situations, for instance), develop a systematic and well-controlled strategy whereby you gradually learn to face up to the stressful situation.
- Get into the habit of identifying your negative thinking and challenging it, while at the same time acting differently. You need both to question your worries and to find alternative, more positive behaviors to help you overcome them.

# pamper yourself in your home spa

When you're in need of rest and recuperation, the ideal is, of course, to escape to a luxurious health spa for the weekend. But if this isn't feasible, or you urgently feel the need to break a cycle of pushing your body to its limits, why not retreat into your own home spa for 48 hours? Turn off the phone, don loose clothing, and spend the weekend cherishing yourself. Believe me, you'll feel revitalized in both mind and body on Monday morning. It can take some people a little longer to feel great—it just depends on how long you've been burning yourself out.

I'd recommend setting at least a weekend aside each season in which to pamper, nurture, and nourish your body. And if you enter these four weekends into your calender months in advance, not only will it prevent you from forgetting this "you" time, but it will also give you some dates to look forward to and remind you to organize everything—and everyone—else so that you can retreat into your sanctuary.

The home spa plan outlined over the following pages is the ideal; if you don't manage it all, it doesn't matter. Relaxing and shifting gear in any way will be beneficial. You also don't need to buy all the foods, teas, oils, and remedies; just select whichever appeal to you and that you think you'll use.

## preparing for a weekend in your home spa

Before embarking on your weekend of rejuvenation, the ideal strategy for luxuriating through a nurturing 48 hours is, a few days beforehand, to stock up on plenty of nutritious foods that will simultaneously cleanse and nourish your body and to treat yourself to a new CD, video, DVD, magazine, or book that has nothing to do with work and everything to do with enjoyment and escapism. However, if your best-laid plans to get ahead don't come to fruition, try to have an early Friday night—no alcohol, favorite chickflick, bath, and then bed, with fresh, clean sheets—and set the alarm for an early-ish start on Saturday morning so that you can get out and stock up on the food and movies, buy flowers, and face packs. (Or you could make your own by mashing a ripe avocado.)

## nourish your body, so your soul feels happy in it

When it comes to nurturing and energizing your body throughout your 48-hour home spa, it's best to give it a small amount of food often, rather than a couple of big meals a day. This is why I've suggested stocking up on plenty of ingredients that you can easily transform into a delicious dish within a few minutes. The best strategy is to have healthful between-meal snacks—seeds, yogurt with fruit, and cheese with fruit—between a yogurt-and-fruit-based breakfast and a protein-rich lunch and supper—perhaps chicken or prosciutto with salad or broiled vegetables for lunch and an omelet with salad for supper—and to follow each meal with fresh fruit.

## bodyfoods 48-hour home spa shopping list

Plenty of fresh fruits and vegetables. Buy fruits that you consider treats, perhaps fresh or frozen summer berries, small fruits, mangoes, cherries, and papayas (which are great diuretics and digestion soothers).

Packaged salad and raw vegetables (ready-peeled ones are fine), ideally organic, to munch on raw, steam, or roast. Celery, fennel, and cucumber are particularly cleansing, as are carrots. Stock up on plenty of carrots, as carrot juice is great for "detox." Buy enough fresh vegetables to provide generous portions for two meals a day.

Some fresh deli soups (but not creamy ones) if you don't feel like making your own.

Avocados to jazz up salads.

Lemons and limes for adding to water to make zingy drinks.

Unsalted nuts and dried fruits (without added sulfur dioxide, $SO_2$), such as figs, apricots, Medjool dates, and mangoes, to snack on.

Lean proteins like eggs, chicken, fish (smoked salmon and gravadlax make hassle-free treats) and lean cold cuts. Buy enough for a couple of meals each day.

Natural organic yogurt and lighter cheeses, such as soft goat cheese, mozzarella, cottage cheese and ricotta. Buy some Parmesan, too—it's high in protein and easy to digest.

Fresh herbs with which to make food tastier (your home-spa weekend should nurture your taste buds, too!). Stock up on fresh mint leaves, in particular, not only for garnishing vegetables with, but also to infuse in boiling water for a herbal tea.

A good-quality virgin olive oil with which to make a simple vinaigrette or to drizzle over broiled vegetables (it's good for your skin, too).

Buy a bottle of vanilla extract to sniff if you think you're going to have a big sugar craving—sniff it whenever you crave sweet foods, and the urge disappears.

If you think you're going to continue to use it afterward, buy a juicing machine—I think they're great, but it can work out expensive if you use it only this weekend. Mind you, once you've tried the real thing and can just feel your juice oozing in nutrients, I bet you won't go back to bottled juices.

# day 1

## morning

*Start your pampering weekend with an invigorating shower, using a stimulating body wash; or you could use few drops of rosemary essential oil on your sponge. Avoid listening to the news; it's usually depressing. Much better to play your favorite music or just enjoy the silence—as this is a luxury.*

*Make a light breakfast such as fruit and yogurt with some fresh juice or water. if you haven't got these ingredients on hand, have as healthful a breakfast as possible—say, a couple of slices of whole-wheat toast with a pure-fruit spread or some cereal, a bagel, or muffin—just something so that you're not going to come over weak while you're running around. Take 350mg milk thistle, ideally before your food, three times a day to help clear out your liver—you'll need to take this every day for the next week.*

*If you haven't had the chance during the week, pop around to your local market or supermarket to stock up on the supplies listed on page 143. Aim to be finished by 12 noon, so that you can then switch the phone off, make yourself something light for lunch, put on some loose, cozy clothes, and shut the door on the outside world, ready to nurture. Note that you may feel a little overemotional while you spa, but just let yourself go through it rather than fighting it. Make a note of the issues it's highlighting, as it would be good to look at them in a few weeks' time when you're feeling more levelheaded to see whether you can resolve them.*

### detox your body with water

Use your spa time to detox your body. Although I'm not convinced of the idea that our bodies contain toxins, I do know that many people feel better after drinking enough water to enable their kidneys to get rid of the unwanted chemicals and byproducts that are circulating in their bodies. Take my advice and you'll certainly feel less toxic and more buoyant. Drink at least 5 pints of water or herbal tea throughout each day. If you're not used to downing this amount, you'll find yourself spending a lot of time on the toilet (take a magazine with you!). Your body will soon adapt to processing these large quantities, however; so your trips to the bathroom will decrease in frequency by the time you return to your normal schedule.

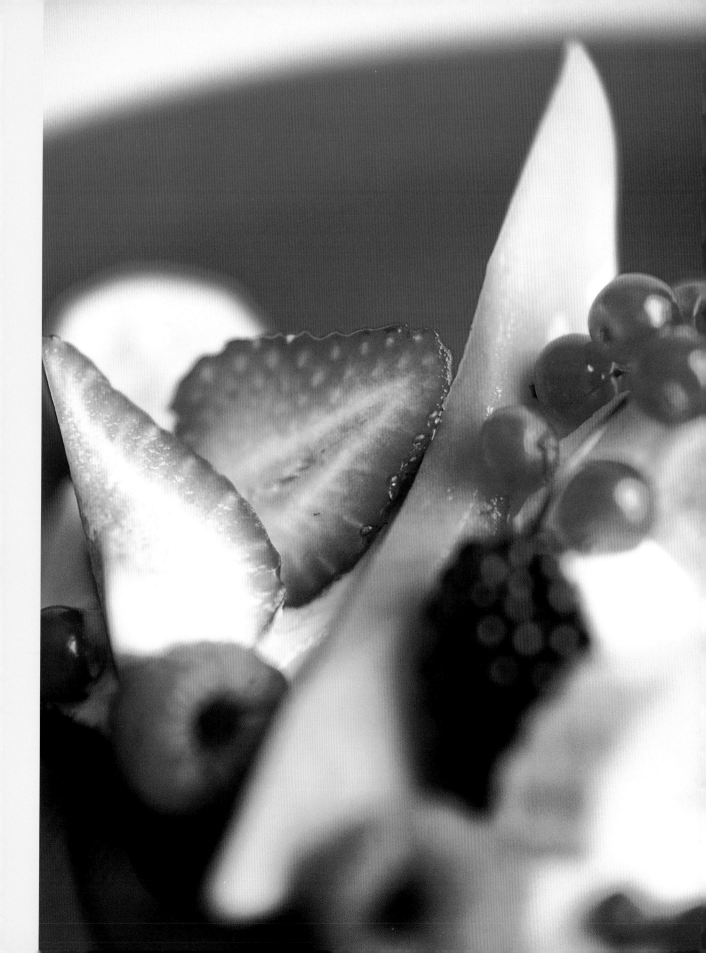

# day 1
## afternoon

*Make some fresh herbal tea such as lemon verbena or camomile (see page 13). Put together a light protein-rich lunch—meat, fish, chicken, a little cheese, lentils, beans, maybe hummus—with plenty of salad or raw vegetables, a fresh juice or a bowl of soup. I've included recipes throughout this 48-hour home spa plan, but numerous dishes in this book are also light and easy to make (try my Roasted Beet and Chicken Salad, on page 23, or Zucchini, Mint, Tomato, and Coriander Seed Salad, on page 118, for example). Carrot juice is great for cleansing, so have a small glass each day—plain or mixed with orange or other vegetables—for the next week. Don't forget to take your milk thistle.*

### AROMATIC FRUIT AND NUT COUSCOUS SALAD (SERVES 1)

Place 3/8 cup couscous in a large bowl and cover with 1/4 cup boiling water. Cover with some plastic wrap and leave to stand for 5 minutes. Meanwhile, heat 1/2 tsp. olive oil in a skillet and fry 1 diced red pepper for 3–4 minutes. Stir in a crushed garlic clove, 1/2 tsp. each ground cumin and coriander and a small pinch of crushed chili flakes, and fry for 1–2 minutes. Next add 1/4 cup roughly chopped pistachio nuts and a generous 1/8 cup finely chopped dates and thoroughly mix through the spicy mix. Peel back the plastic wrap from the couscous and fluff up the grains with a fork. Stir in the spicy fruit and nut mixture and add a small handful of roughly torn mint. Season to taste, then eat immediately while still warm.

*Follow lunch with some fruit. After an hour or so of relaxing, try the exercises opposite. Rebeca Nonika, a physical therapist and cranial osteopath, has worked wonders with overly busy, stressed-out clients of mine by teaching them to exercise in ways that feel natural to the body. I've included some of her exercises that would be great to do in your home spa—I find them wonderfully relaxing when I'm overwrought or need to ground and re-energize myself. Because your body might be unused to exercising, or just drained on a Saturday, do only gentle, warm-up exercises. Once you've worked through them, spend the rest of the afternoon lounging around until it's time to exercise some more. Have a fruit snack, fresh or dried, or some unsalted nuts an hour before exercising again to keep up your blood-sugar level.*

Lying on your bed, stretch both arms above your head and take a deep breath. This will help to put you in a positive frame of mind.

Lying on your side, bring up both heels toward your buttocks. Then, keeping your legs together, swing them to one side and then to the other.

Roll from one side of the bed to the other to get your side muscles moving.

Lying on your tummy, bend one knee, straighten it so that you stretch out your leg, then lift your leg to strengthen your buttock muscles. Repeat this with your other leg.

Get out of bed and perform a standing stretch by stretching your arms above your head. Clasping both hands together, now bend to your right and then to your left.

Still in the same position, turn to your right and then to your left.

To help to keep your balance, hold on to something. Now with your knee straight, stretch one leg to the side, backward and then forward as far as you can, all the while maintaining an upright position.

Repeat with your other leg.

Balancing on your toes, and then your heels, move up and down. Now walk a few steps on your toes, and then on your heels.

Perform some mini-squats with your knees apart (similar to a skiing posture).

Perform some circles with your arms as if you were doing the crawl in a swimming pool.

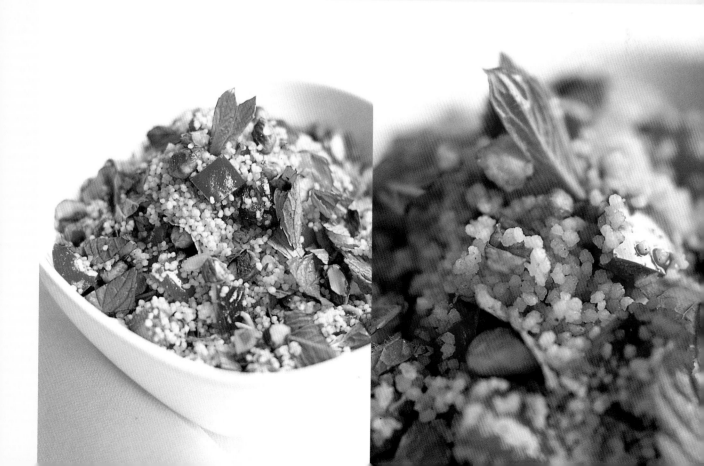

# day 1 evening

*The early evening is the time for some abdominal and relaxation exercises.*

- Lying on your back, raise each leg in turn above your tummy, keeping your stomach muscles contracted (as if you were pulling your navel toward your back).

- In the same position, repeat step 1 with both legs together, but don't lower them to rest this time. Keep the range of this movement very short, as if you were performing crunches.

- Standing upright, bend to the side, then make a small arc up and down again. Repeat this movement 30 times, gently returning to the center. Change sides and repeat the process.

- On all fours (as if you were a cat), stretch both arms forward and sit on your heels. This gives your back a long stretch.

- Still in the cat position, stretch both arms forward to the left and then forward to the right.

- Again in the cat position, stretch your right arm forward and your left leg backward. Then stretch your left arm forward and your right leg backward.

- Lying on your back, relax your neck by gently tucking your chin downward, toward the floor, taking care not to strain your neck muscles.

- Still lying down, relax your back and neck and focus on feeling the contact that your body is making with the floor. Starting with your heels, and working inch by inch toward your head, relax all of the areas that are still tense.

## relaxing oils to take the body into the nuturing, slow-breathing zone

*Use just a few drops of any of the following, as too much can actually turn them into stimulants.*

- vetiver
- lavender
- geranium
- lemon
- camomile
- clary sage
- marjoram
- rose

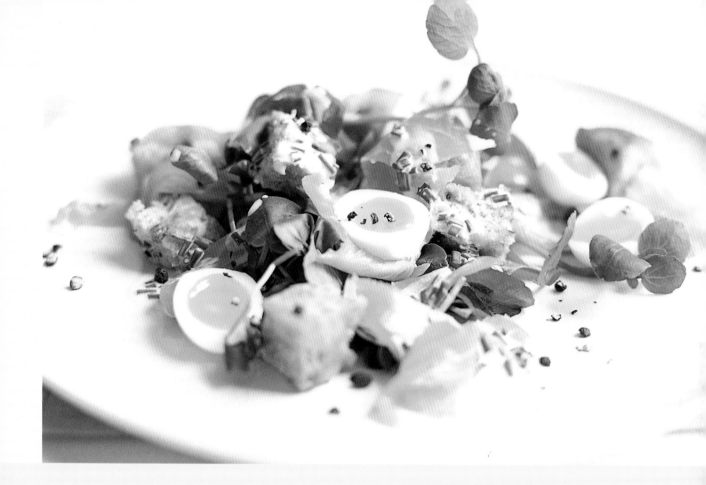

*Once you've exercised and bathed, choose a meal that is light and quick to prepare. My Smoked Salmon and Egg Salad is a real luxury.*

## SMOKED SALMON AND EGG SALAD (SERVES 1)

First heat 1 Tbs. olive oil in a large skillet, and add some bread cubes cut from 1 slice of seed bread. Fry until lightly golden and crisp. Remove from the pan and leave to drain on a paper towel. Bring a small pan of water to the boil, then carefully drop in 3 quail eggs. Leave to gently simmer for exactly 3 minutes, then, using a spoon, carefully drop them into a bowl of iced water and leave to cool. If you can't find quail eggs, use a chicken egg, boiled and cut into quarters. Meanwhile, make a quick lemon and chive dressing. Spoon 1 Tbs. mayonnaise into a small bowl and stir in the juice and zest from ½ lemon. Thin the mayonnaise down further with a little water to make into a pourable dressing, then add 1 Tbs. snipped chives and season to taste. Arrange a few arugula leaves and watercress leaves on a serving plate. Lay rough strips of 2½ oz. smoked salmon and the peeled and halved or quartered eggs on top. Drizzle the dressing over the salad and sprinkle with the croutons. Serve immediately.

*Sometimes your digestive system can become unsettled and bloated when you stop and have a big change to your diet, in which case drink plenty of fresh mint tea to help settle it down.*

# day 2
## morning

First thing, infuse some lemon slices in a large pot of hot water and drink to help clear your system out. Remember to take your milk thistle. Now make a light breakfast, choosing from the following: fruit, yogurt sprinkled with roasted seeds, a smoothie, cold meats, cheese, eggs (scrambled or boiled), perhaps a light lentil soup, or maybe some miso soup with seaweed.

### energizing oil blends for exercising

Burn the following oil blend while exercising. You could also use this blend to revive you after your post-exercise shower. If your muscles are unused to the exercise and start to ache, try soaking in a bath with thyme essential oil and, once you've dried off, rubbing any aching areas gently with Arnica cream (don't use on broken skin).

- **4** drops rosemary
- **8** drops eucalyptus or peppermint
- **5** drops lavender
- **7** drops grapefruit

At least an hour after eating, the morning is the time to start stretching your whole body. Put on loose, comfortable clothing, switch off the phone, put on some music, and shut the door on the outside world.

1 Bend forward and try to reach as low as you can.

2 Perform a full squat, keeping your heels on the ground (if necessary, hold on to something).

3 Stretch your body by taking a big step backward and trying to put your heel on the ground. Repeat this procedure with your other leg.

4 Take a step to the left, transfer your weight to your right leg and then stretch the inner part of your left leg by squatting on your right, weight-bearing leg. Now stretch your right leg in the same way.

5 Standing upright, stretch the front muscles of your left thigh by placing your heel on your buttock.

6 Repeat, using your right leg.

7 Swing your hips from side to side and then around and around.

8 For some gentle neck exercises, look to the ceiling and then to the ground; turn your head from side to side, then cock your head to the left, so that your ear is resting on your shoulder, and then to the right.

9 Imagine that someone is pulling the crown of your head upward, in line with your spine, and elongate your spine to improve your posture.

10 Take a deep breath as you raise both shoulders; now breathe out and lower both shoulders, as if you were unloading a heavy weight.

11 Shake your arms, and with them your body, as if you were shaking off sand from the beach.

*Spend the rest of the morning relaxing, then make a light lunch. If you're ravenous, nibble on raw vegetables, fresh fruits and dried roasted seeds. Remember to drink your water, herbal tea, or a small glass of carrot juice, or make your own energizing fruit juice.*

## ZINGY RUBY GRAPEFRUIT AND PASSION-FRUIT JUICE (SERVES 1)

Place the seeds and flesh of 4 passion fruits (the seeds make this juice slightly crunchy) and the flesh of 1 large ruby grapefruit in a blender and blend until smooth. Alternatively, push the passion-fruit pulp through a sieve before blending it with the grapefruit. If you prefer a gentler fruit hit, try making my peach and strawberry juice with 1 large, ripe peach, a small orange, and a handful of strawberries. Remove the stone from the peach, place its flesh in a blender, along with the freshly squeezed orange juice and strawberries, and blend away. Add some ice cubes for a cool drink.

*If the weather's sunny, some great ways of nourishing your body are to start the day with an invigorating walk in the park, to have breakfast on your balcony or patio, or simply to bask at a window that catches the sun. Our bodies need to be safely exposed to the sun's ultraviolet rays because they encourage the skin to produce vitamin D, a nutrient that's essential for maintaining the health of the bones, muscles, and immune system. So protect it with sunscreen and light clothing, but let your skin luxuriate in the sunshine.*

*and let the sun shine!*

# day 2
## afternoon

*Make yourself a light lunch, such as my Oriental Noodle Salad.*

### ORIENTAL NOODLE SALAD (SERVES 1)

Bring a large pan of water to the boil and drop in 1 sheet of egg noodles. Leave to simmer for 3 minutes or according to the package instructions, then drain well. Meanwhile, finely shred 2 green onions, 2/3 cup snow peas and 1/2 large carrot into very thin lengths and transfer them to a large serving bowl. Add a handful of beansprouts and the noodles, and toss through the vegetables. Meanwhile, make a dressing by whisking together 1 tsp. freshly grated ginger, 1 small crushed garlic clove, the zest and juice from 1/2 lime, 1/2 tsp. sugar, 2 tsp. sesame oil, and 2 tsp. fish sauce. Drizzle this over the salad, and scatter a small handful of roughly torn cilantro leaves and 2 tsp. toasted sesame seeds on top.

*If your body yearns for a snooze after your lunch, give in to it, but if you feel like some light exercise, you have a choice. You could either repeat the exercises that you did on day 1 or, if you prefer something more calming, try this breathing exercise. Once you have mastered it, you can use it when you're stuck in the middle of a manic day or on a plane, or when you're waiting for a meeting to start. Do a few rounds of this complete-breathing exercise—you'll be amazed how dramatically your adrenaline and stress levels drop and how quickly your mind becomes clear and focused. As you gradually acquire the habit of complete breathing, your method of respiration will also slowly, but surely, improve.*

*Before you begin, burn some relaxing oils, such as lavender or jasmine. To start, familiarize yourself with this exercise by lying comfortably on your back, perhaps on a rug or fluffy towel. It is important to train yourself to concentrate entirely on the action of breathing, which means forcing yourself to empty your mind of the random thoughts and to-do lists that will inevitably be swirling around it.*

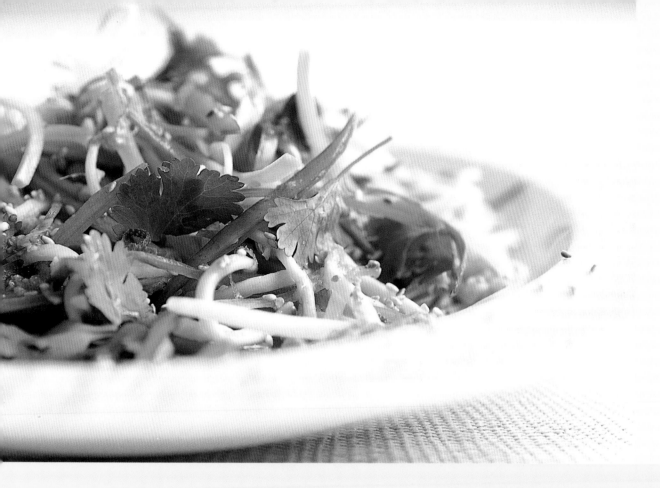

1 Empty your lungs completely by breathing out.

2 Slowly lower your diaphragm, allowing air to enter your lungs. When your abdomen swells, filling the

3 bottom of your lungs with air, then…

4 Expand your ribs without straining them, then…

Allow your lungs to fill completely by raising your shoulder blades.

5 When your lungs are completely full, breathe out as you did in step 1.

6 Now breathe in again in the same way as steps 2–4.

*Throughout this procedure, the air should enter your lungs in a continuous flow. Don't gasp or make any noise. This is an anytime, anyplace exercise, which is why it is essential to learn to perform it silently. You can repeat these steps as often as you wish—they shouldn't induce any discomfort or fatigue. Whenever you feel tired, depressed, or discouraged, do a few complete-breathing exercises and your fatigue will disappear, your mental balance will be restored, and you'll be able to set to work again with renewed vigor.*

*After doing your exercises, be they complete-breathing or otherwise, have some freshly squeezed juice. You could stroll to your local health-food store or deli to buy some. Better still, make your own (see page 151).*

# day 2

## evening

Make a light protein-, vegetable-, and fruit-rich supper, then drink a large mug of relaxing herbal tea. It's now a good time to reevaluate where you're at, having spent the weekend destressing, and take some time to think about how you can avoid becoming so stressed in the future. I also suggest you take a few notes or copy key phrases to carry around with you in your handbag to read on the bus or subway, or stuck in a traffic jam, or when you have a couple of minutes to spare. Destressing is like learning to ride a bike–you'll manage for a minute to stay on course, then wobble and fall off; but the wise thing is to read your notes again and get back on. Eventually you will remember them, and, hopefully find you're a lot less angst-ridden than before. Take advantage of the final hours of your home spa by burning some relaxing oils, sipping herbal tea and visualizing calm.

## evening oils to take you down to deep relaxation
These oils are also good in self-hypnosis and meditation.

- rose Maroc
- jasmine
- vanilla
- hyacinth
- valerian
- narcissus

## visualization

Try this visualization exercise to help you relax: sit comfortably (having turned off the phone, including your cellphone—something I love to do). Close your eyes and imagine you're on a desert island. Use your senses to explore the sights, sounds, and smells as you drift deeper into a beautiful, relaxed meditative state. Stay like this for as long as you like; then, when you're ready, bring your awareness back to the present, safe in the knowledge that you can retreat to this desert, this zone, whenever and wherever you choose. This is a good relaxation exercise to use if you're having a panic attack or experiencing difficulty getting to sleep.

## readjusting to normal life

For the week after this spa weekend, try to keep up as many of the good habits—the drinking water (if you're missing coffee or tea, see pages 24–5 for advice as to how to enjoy it), taking the milk thistle, eating plenty of fresh fruits and vegetables, focusing on proteins and light food, but incorporate some whole grains, such as whole-wheat bread, pasta, and cereals; perhaps start the day off with granola or porridge, or add some rice or potatoes (stick to steamed or boiled, rather than fried or anything creamy or heavy) to your main meals. Keep exercising. And "remembering to breathe out as well as in" is a phrase I use when I find it all becoming a little too much. Food-wise, you may find that your body feels more energetic and lighter if you stick to a high-protein, low-starch lunch, but then eat your relaxing starches, the pasta, rice etc., in the evening. Keep food as light as possible, for if you suddenly go out and eat a rich, fatty, or sugary meal after you've been spa-ing, you will probably end up with bellyache and feel dreadful. Ideally, you will feel so much better that you'll ask yourself why you would ever go back to your own not-so-great habits.

## body-friendly tactics for a stress-free work environment

- Take a few minutes at the beginning of each day to think ahead to food times, so that you can grab something healthful from home, pick up a few nutritious bits on the way to work, or, if you're lucky enough to have a secretary, ask him/her to order some healthful foods to fit in with your day, so that you're not reliant on last-minute snack foods.
- Carry a small bottle of mineral water around with you, so that you can stay hydrated, clearer-minded, and less likely to feel stressed.
- Keep some energizing fruit in your handbag, on your desk, and in meetings, along with water, instead of relying on the usual tea, coffee, and cookies, which have few plus points.
- Put some flowers on your desk or in your meeting room to inspire you and your colleagues.
- Dissipate stress as soon as you feel anxiety levels rising by massaging the kidney area (the soft area of your lower and middle back) in a circular motion, using your fists. This can be done secretly. Friends and patients of mine swear by its effects.
- Keep a stock of relaxing herbal teas at work (see page 13), valerian being one of the best. Bach Mimulus Original Flower Remedy is a good one to carry around.

# index

# acknowledgments

Without my wonderful family—both young and, as we've come to realize, not so young—and treasured friends Navin, David, Caroline, Will, Oliver, Allan, Angelika, Sylvie, Cat, "little Si," Sarah and Peter, Sharon, Anthony, Katingo, Dimiti, Martin, Toni, Bill, Susie, Brett, Emily, Jonas, Barnaby, Susan, Sarah, Peter, Clemance, Cedrick, Shah, Luna, Armina, Rupa, Helen, Nigel, Bea, Brian, Allegra, Charles, Brigitte, Leisha, Mary, Scott, Tony and Angela Immy, Margaret, Bill, Monty, Luna, Anthony, Diane, and Gil, I would never have managed to keep smiling, nor laughed nor cried enough to remain clear-headed and able to write this book. I owe you all everything.

Special thanks to Clare Haworth-Maden, who has been a tower of strength, and to Signora Tetta, who made Italy a culinary haven and inspired me to keep cooking. Tessa Graham, Tara Donovan, Danny McCubbin, Matt Ubter, Jamie Oliver, Chris Terry, Lisa Sullivan, Mike Frost, Louise Holland, Les Cullen, Sara Emslie, Georgia Katz, Rebecca Nonika Borra Garson, Michelle Wadsley, Jane O'Shea, Lisa Pendreigh, Rachel Atkins, Clare Lewis, Jeremy Cogle, and last, but by no means least, Mark Higginbottom, have all helped to keep me on the straight and narrow (no easy task!) by working their butts off, for which I'm extremely grateful.